T0029613

Advance praise for *Between Rock and a Hard Place*

"Between Rock and a Hard Place" is as fine a Montana memoir as I've read in a long time. Maggie Anderson's long goodbye to Rock's slow descent into Parkinson's disease is shaped by hard written edges: an abiding love of the wild land and all the creatures who live there, loyalty, betrayal and the kind of anger you might see peering out from the edge of a badger hole. It's also a stern indictment of our medical establishment. Maggie's courage is as strong as her heart. I can't wait for more from this writer."
—Doug Peacock, author of *Was it Worth it?*, National Outdoor Book Award winner

"Maggie Anderson's powerful memoir reads like a thriller, taking us on a roller coaster ride of hope and despair as Maggie and her husband Rockey journey from the heaven of Montana's rugged backcountry to the hell of Rockey's increasingly disabling Parkinson's Disease. As Rockey slowly loses his body and mind to the disease, and his behavior is warped by pain and desperation, Maggie remains by his side, his steadfast companion and fierce advocate who navigates this sinking ship with strength, grace, and a generosity of spirit that is truly inspirational. This is a gripping and brutally honest memoir of love and loss that will keep you on the edge of your seat from the first page to the last."
—Elise Atchison, author of *Crazy Mountain*

"Love is hard. In this bracing memoir, Maggie Anderson takes the full measure of it—where it comes from, how it pumps the blood, and, heartbreakingly, how she clung to it, alone, as her beloved Rockey left her by increments, caught in an illness that couldn't be turned back or moderated, only endured. Maggie endured to the other side of something she never wanted, finding out what else love is. It's making a place for yourself in the corners where time and tide toss you, insisting on life beyond the wreckage."
—Craig Lancaster, author of *And It Will Be a Beautiful Life*

"*Between Rock and a Hard Place* pulls no punches in describing the harrowing physical and emotional toll a debilitating disease takes on both victim and caretaker. Anderson's take is wry, stoic, and at times, laugh-out-loud funny. A compelling read."
—Gwen Florio, author of *Silent Hearts*

"A work of great strength, honesty, and compassion. This is an important book and you will be better equipped for life after reading it."
—Daniel J. Rice, author of *The Unpeopled Season*

Between Rock and a
Hard Place

a memoir

Maggie Anderson

Riverfeet Press
Livingston, MT
Bemidji, MN
Abingdon, VA
www.riverfeetpress.com

Between Rock and a Hard Place: A Memoir
Non-fiction/Memoir/Health/Adventure
Copyright 2023 © by the author
All rights reserved.
ISBN-13: 979-8985398830
LCCN: 2022941373

This title is available at a special discount to booksellers and libraries. Send inquiries to: riverfeetpress@gmail.com

This book is dedicated to the one and only Rockey Goertz. For the love and laughs. For the lessons in courage and moving forward, always forward and for all the adventures, and for inadvertently teaching me to bring my best self every day.

Between Rock and a

Hard Place

a memoir

Maggie Anderson

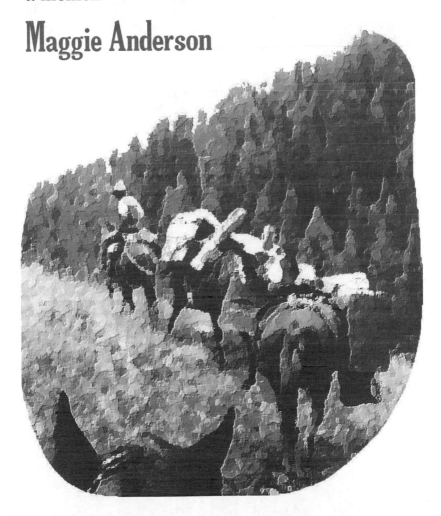

Prelude

The mountain pack trips were our favorite adventures and we most often explored the mountains of the Gallatin Range in Montana. Before we moved to the Treasure State permanently, we would haul five or six horses and mules from Minnesota and pack into mountains for as long as we could stay.

Making lists, gathering supplies, laying out our cold weather gear—where are those damn good boots? We'd lay all these things out on the floor of wherever we were staying and check the piles against the lists. Something in me liked the order of this process, maybe because so much of these trips was a little risky, physically demanding and always chaotic as we loaded the pack mules and mounted up on our own horses and left the trailhead.

After laying it all out and rechecking the lists, we would divide the loads into piles that each animal would carry. The biggest concern was keeping each side of each animal's packs evenly weighted. So after we settled on the piles for each mule, we weighed the contents and shifted things around until the weight was evenly distributed. Rockey was a wizard at this. He could remember the weight of the pan set and the cots, the weight of a 12-pack of beer or the portable stove from year to year, so the piles were nearly perfect and required only shuffling a couple of things around. From these piles, we loaded everything into the packs for three pack mules. Berta the giant, kindest mule carried the most weight and the most awkward load. She had the wall tent, its aluminum poles, some odd-shaped PVC structures that held fishing gear and stove parts. That stuff was on top of the Super Packs—big, hard-plastic packs that were custom made to fit the curve of her body and held 125 pounds per side with pots and pans, most of the food, lanterns, an axe and dozens of other necessities. The kitchen boxes were the lightest and the easiest to load. Custom-made heavy-gauge aluminum packs that when taken apart could be made into a workspace that held the stove, some shelving and a prep area for cooking. A dainty red mule named Reba was the only one who could manage the compact kitchen boxes. The clanging and banging drove many a mule to come undone, scattering contents everywhere. Reba was a kitchen-hauling rockstar as she trudged along on her tiny hooves carrying her noisy business. The third packer was a small red mule named Ruby. She wasn't nice, but she did a good job with the third load packed in orange plastic pack boxes consisting of a table, chairs, a cook tent, floor tarp, high lines, horse feed, stove and pipes. Rockey, strong and tall, did all the heavy lifting of the packs onto the mules as I scurried underneath tying knots and securing buckles. Nothing about Rockey's elk camp prep was lacking in either details or comforts. Eventually, I became a pretty good packer, but it was only after lots of these trips and loading up under Rockey's watchful eye that I felt I could have done it by myself.

In addition to the loads the pack mules carried, we had gear on our own horses, piled high behind the saddle: our clothes, toiletries, extra-warm clothes and sleeping bags. It took a big swing of a right leg to clear the height on those cantle packs.

The mornings when we left the trailhead for camp were full of anxiety for me, and I could hardly breathe by the time we finally got loaded and heading up the trail. I would picture every disaster possible from rolling off cliffs to being swept away in a creek before we even got mounted. Thankfully, about a mile into the ten-mile ride, I'd look around and see all the majesty of the country we were headed into and the worries would fall away. This is when the part I loved started to kick in. Rockey, perpetually serene in the wilderness, always led the string of mules while I covered the back. My job was to watch the packs for slippage and to maintain a steady pace to push the string along. I liked being back there all by myself. Miles of stunning vistas, no talking, in and out of dark forests and open meadows, crossing creek after creek, always heading up and up toward that ridgeline in my faraway vision and rarely seeing another human. Riding the back was the easiest part, and I savored every step of the slow climb to the high meadow we would call home for a few weeks.

It took about four and a half hours to reach the big meadow where we set up camp. The spot was a bowl, or cirque, with a sparkling fresh creek at the edge. There was a steep and rocky high ridgeline on three sides and the meadow was lush with tall green grasses sloped gently downhill toward the trail we'd just ridden. From the top of that ridge, we could look down into Paradise Valley far off in the east.

First things first, when we arrived we tied the mules and horses. The saddle horses only got their cinches released a little while they stood quietly and rested. The hurry-up part came in unloading the mules and their heavy packs. After untying a couple dozen knots and unlatching another dozen buckles, they were free of their burdens. A log we had moved on a prior trip was always still in its place and that's where we laid all the saddles and tack up off the ground, covered with tarps. Once we got both mules and horses unpacked, unsaddled and watered, Rock would dig out his beer to set in the cold creek and look for the table and chairs. I always made a beeline for the coffee pot and tiny gas stove to get some coffee cooking. We'd just unpack enough to sit down before we set up the tent, took a deep breath and took in the incredible beauty of the place we had worked so hard to get to. I can still close my eyes and remember the feeling of absolute peace I found in the silence of that place. The memory of it is so sweet to me.

We made a camp in this wondrous place for many years in a row. The days of those high backcountry camps left a mark on me and a different mark on Rockey, I suppose. He was always looking for something. Elk sign or elk or which way they were traveling or where he would sit in his scentless camouflage hunting clothes to have a good archery shot, should he get lucky. For me it was more about just looking and feeling. Everything was different up there. The air was thinner and crisp feeling on my skin. I would make a small dam with rocks from the cold creek, so we'd have a tiny pool to collect water for the day and always remember to water the horses and mules downstream from our collection pool.

We would sometimes hike the ridge of the bowl together, both watchful and alert, but looking for totally different things. I looked for plants, bear sign and watched hopefully for goats. The views of the Madison Range far off to the west made my heart skip a beat every time we climbed up. It was a lucky day if I saw some bear sign or found a weird sea fossil at somewhere around 9,000 feet. Rock saw everything, but he only looked for elk tracks or scat or yesterday's bed. Maybe he loved the air up there too and surely loved the silence like I did. But I always wondered if he craved the single-mindedness of his time in that magical place.

Days in camp had a simplicity that felt like a balm to our work-rattled spirits. Wake up, check the horses, stoke the stove, get some wood for the fire and some water for coffee and a morning toilette. Start the coffee, water the horses, maybe grab some wood. We would each get a big mug of coffee—I even had real cream for it—and each grab a couple of horses and lead them out to the meadow to graze for a bit. Sweet-smelling grass sparkled with light frost and the horses greedily grabbing their breakfast making soft chewing sounds with only an occasional snort or snuffle. It was another slice of the beloved silence of the wilderness and the calm of grazing horses.

After the ponies were satisfied, we'd feed ourselves. Meals in the backcountry always tasted better and we always ate well in our camp. Bacon, eggs, fried potatoes and toast with a few more cups of excellent camp coffee for breakfast. Then some simple and necessary work: more wood, heat water to wash dishes, check the horses, look around with binoculars and think of another adventure.

On days we didn't hike far, we would saddle up two horses and leave the others tied in camp and ride around exploring the rises and curves of the forest away from camp. I once found a rock as big as my living room encrusted with thousands of ocean fossils. It was almost too big a thought to know that oceans had once covered this high place. Rockey enjoyed the sights and smells, and he looked for elk. The late day was a repeat of the morning rituals with wood, fire, water and food for all. Sometimes we played cribbage at night by the stove in our wall tent lit with the soft yellow light of lanterns. Most often, we dragged our chairs outside and listened to the night sounds. Clattering rocks above us let us know the goats were here. Elk bugles and peeps from an out-of-sight meadow sometimes silenced by wolves howling. If the conditions were right, meaning not too dry, we would make a small campfire and sit snugly in our chairs with feet propped up on the fire's circle of rocks. Camp boots always had some melted parts on them.

First Sign
2002

It was mid-April when we left the Dudley Creek cabin near Big Sky, heading back to the farm in Minnesota after the last day of the ski season. Rockey was a skilled downhill skier and snowboarder. This year he chose to ride his board and we had spent over fifty days on the mountain during the ski season.

In February, his two adult sons, Nick and Rock Jr had come for a visit and they rode every day that week. I skipped a day of boarding in the middle of their stay. They all went up to Moonlight Basin and hiked the ridge to find some good powder and serious vertical. They had a blast, making runs as fast as they could … something about most vertical feet for the price of a lift ticket. Other than red faces flushed with cold and the joy of flying down the mountain, they reported nothing unusual about the day.

Later that night, as we lay in bed, Rockey said, "I fell today." An occasion that called for a little ribbing, as one of the givens in the snowboard world of Rockey Goertz is that he never falls. He said he jammed his shoulder in what they refer to as a "yard sale" fall. He fell hard enough to lose his helmet and spin spread eagle, face down almost a hundred feet, tearing off both gloves and coming unclipped from his board before he stuck his arm out to stop himself from slamming into a tree. Other than his shoulder feeling stiff, he didn't think he'd hurt anything more than his pride. He even cracked a smile I could see in the moonlight streaming through the windows when he told me how hard his kids had laughed. Just a regular day on the mountain with good snow, blue skies and lots of belly laughs. Except laying there in the moonlight after Rockey drifted off to sleep, I thought how odd it was that it wasn't his first fall that season. There had been others when it was just the two of us. None of those tumbles were as dramatic as today's, but it quietly passed through my conscious thought that he had fallen more than once that year.

In April, after Big Sky closed for the season, on the long drive back to Minnesota, with the dogs and our luggage in the back of the Expedition, we listened to good music and audio books. Rockey was a super talkative guy when life was good, and he had business or personal adventures to plan. We'd been talking about wrapping up the last few homes in a residential development and opening the last phase of another, when I asked, "What's the deal with that thumb twitch? I've noticed it's been going on for a while." He looked at his left hand draped over the steering wheel and we both watched his thumb dance in a rhythmic way. He replied that he thought it was from the big fall in February and that maybe he had pinched a nerve in that twisting, turning, jamming tumble. I said I didn't think a two-month twitch was reasonable and maybe he should get it looked at. He agreed, and we resumed our chair dancing and rocking out to Bob Seeger singing as the miles flew by.

As June gave way to July, the thumb twitch appeared to be gaining intensity, now involving the index finger of his left hand. When I reminded him about getting it checked, he asked me to make an appointment to see a neurologist, which I did after we came home from our late summer pack trip.

9

Sometime in early fall of 2002, Rockey and I made our way down the halls of a local hospital to wait in blue hospital chairs outside the office of a neurologist.

I don't remember this doctor's name, but he was quick to render his clinical diagnosis. This refers to a diagnosis that is made by observing symptoms, performing a few noninvasive neurological tests and taking the patient's medical history. He asked about previous surgeries, existing conditions, medications, and general health questions. After about a quarter of an hour, he pronounced that "In my opinion you have Parkinson's disease, Mr. Goertz."

He didn't seem to open the door for many questions but handed us a piece of paper with a name and phone number, saying, "Call Dr. T at the University of Minnesota Hospital and make an appointment to get a second opinion." He would send the referral.

On the heels of this doctor visit, I made the appointment with Dr. T for a week from that day. After an internet search, I learned that Parkinson's was difficult to diagnose and often misdiagnosed because of the lack of lab tests available to confirm it. It turned out that Dr. T specialized in movement disorders, primarily Parkinson's Disease, and he had led years of research into the mysterious affliction. Again, with the long hospital hallways and blue hospital chairs in front of a curved station where a dozen or so personnel directed patients down yet some other distant hallway. We were called back and found Dr. T, a soft-spoken yet intense man. He was deft at including me in the conversation but leaving no doubt that Rockey was his patient. In all the years that were to follow, there was never again a doctor who treated Rockey with such calm patience and compassion as Dr T. He spent over an hour asking questions and performing more involved clinical tests. He watched him walk down a long hallway and asked me questions about Rockey's gait and movement, pointing out the things that he was seeing. A small head tilt, the tiniest hint of a left foot slowness. We went back to his small, cluttered office and he had Rock sit in a chair facing him. More tests ensued. Lots of finger tapping other fingers, faster, slower. Then tapping feet, right then left, fast then slow. His diagnosis was the same, but Dr. T then explained that Parkinson's was a degenerative disorder of the central nervous system that mainly affects the motor system. We heard for the first time about the part of the brain called the substantia nigra and dopamine production, or more precisely, the fact that Rockey's brain would eventually cease producing dopamine, a neurotransmitter vital to the transmission of information between nerve cells in the brain. He told us about agonists and levodopa to treat the symptoms that Rockey would be facing. When Rockey asked, "Well, how do you fix it?" the doctor kindly replied, "There is no cure. It always gets worse."

As our heads reeled with the overload of information, I remember him saying that Rockey was lucky/unlucky. Lucky because he was fit, strong and physically active, but unlucky because he was being diagnosed at just fifty years old, and that put him into the class of early onset Parkinson's. There was less research completed on early onset so hence, little understanding of the progression Rockey would face. He also said Rockey would likely be in a wheelchair within ten years.

I don't have many specific recollections of the time that followed that day. I know I stayed up late for a week, reading pages and pages of information on Parkinson's and the treatments commonly prescribed. I began to form an understanding of the medical jargon that Dr. T had used. I found who was doing research and what kinds of studies they were working on. I printed hundreds of pages of opinions, drug protocols and clinical trials. I cried for hours as I scrolled through the pages filled with words I had to look up to try to understand what this disease was going to do to Rockey. I made pile after pile of papers about Parkinson's. By the end of my research period, I had a thick three-ring binder full of information that I would take in during the overnight hours of the coming weeks. That day and for the duration of his life, I became the researcher, information gatherer and fierce advocate for Rockey, a role he depended on as his body gradually failed him.

. . .

On this day, Rockey quit talking. He went to work at what I called the House Factory – building custom homes in the northern suburbs of St. Paul. He came home and did farm work like we did every day. Summer held a never-ending list of farm tasks. We baled several hundred acres of hay with typically three cuts per season. We grew corn and had a herd of cattle. There was always work to be done, from equipment or fence repairs to one of the many steps in harvesting the crops. We ate late supper and watched TV without speaking. Without having to ask, I knew his silence had nothing to do with me, so I simply lived with it. I spoke minimally in those following days but told him things about my job or the horses and cows or the count of hay bales we had for the coming winter. I asked if he'd like some cake. I knew him well enough to understand that he was processing the doctor's words, and when he was ready, he'd let me know.

A couple of weeks went by before he came into the house at the end of the day and said, "Okay, I'm ready to talk about it."

I asked, "So, what did you come up with?"

I sat down in the big, open living room and Rockey leaned against the twelve-foot wide, tumbled brick fireplace that he and his partner Tim built one hot, shirtless, beer-filled summer weekend. He began with, "I decided that I'll have plenty of time later to feel sorry for myself, so I'm done with that. I want to keep doing what I'm doing, just maybe a little faster." He talked about the upcoming presentations he needed to make before the Lino Lakes City Council to get final approval for the last phase of a residential housing development. He explained that his tremor got worse when he was feeling stressed, so he wanted to get his head right to keep from tremoring visibly before the council. Those meetings were incredibly stressful because they were often contentious and the outcome, no matter what, had a huge financial impact on his and Tim's company. He was afraid the tremor would diminish him in the eyes of the council. Rockey had a long history of successful residential developments in the northern St. Paul suburbs and enjoyed his reputation as the big silver-haired guy who got things done to the city's satisfaction. He was living the life of *local boy does good*.

I wasn't surprised that he included completing this project in his decisions about how to deal with his diagnosis. He had a way of thinking that was clear and sharp, laying out scenarios and rolling around in potential outcomes. He went on to say that we should probably get busy on some more of the adventures we'd been dreaming of.

I asked him how he felt about the diagnosis. As he started to pace from the fireplace to me, he spoke with animation and he yelled, "How do you think I feel?"

I waited until he walked back to the fireplace, and I softly said, "I don't know, Rock, but I wish you would tell me." He stared at me, and I quietly continued, "Are you angry? Are you scared … depressed?"

He started walking again and said too loudly, "Yes I'm mad! And I'm fucking scared!" I got up, walked to him and stood on tiptoes and wrapped my arms around him. Rock was a little over 6'3" and if I stood tall, I was 5'5". I stroked his hair and held him tight, and we began to weep. He quietly said, "I'm so, so sad, I can hardly stand it." We stood there for a long time as he wept in my arms. I believe we both had unspoken thoughts about what our future might be.

Rockey's Story

Rockey was one of those guys who could do anything. We first crossed paths in the late 80s, and at the time we were both in our late thirties. I thought he had the world by the ass and so did he. He was a successful home builder and contractor with a great business partner, Tim Klosner, who was also his best friend. At over six-foot-three, Rockey had plenty of early silver hair, the ropey upper body muscles of a working man, thickly muscled legs from marathon running and a smile that could light up the night. He was an accomplished, exuberant skier and snowboarder who loved the thrill of steep and deep. Forests of the Upper Midwest and the wilderness of the northern Rocky Mountains spoke to his heart when he hiked and rode horseback looking for promising deer and elk habitat. As a true Harley guy, he rode big and far, often alone, and kept the shiny side up for over thirty years.

In our early life together, Rock was devoted to growing his companies and replenishing his coffers after his divorce. He paid a reasonable price for a one-hundred-acre parcel in North Branch, Minnesota, from a wealthy friend and mentor, and began his life as a farmer. Over the next few years, the companies thrived, and his farm grew to over five hundred acres. He worked long days at his jobs and endless hours on the farm, growing hay and corn and raising beef cattle. Still, we had time for some grand adventures. I owned an advertising and marketing company and was able to keep a flexible schedule sometimes. Farming and building homes shared the same off-season, which made for some memorable ski and snowboard vacations. Every year starting at Thanksgiving, he took his sons Rock Jr. and Nick, along with his partner Tim and Tim's son Wally, and headed for Big Sky. There, in the early season, they would shred the mountain, doing all the steepest and nastiest runs over and over until Christmas. The rest of the winter he and I visited the Gallatin Valley in Montana, often making the 1,100-mile drive from Minnesota in fourteen and a half hours, skiing and snowboarding until our legs were weak.

Everything about Rockey was opposed to moderation. He worked hard and long hours. When he wasn't working, he played hard for long hours. His attitude was one of great optimism and enthusiasm for whatever the day brought him. If we were cleaning the barn and paddocks, it would be, "We'll be done in no time!" When he was selling new homes out of a model home, the hours ran from 5:00 p.m. to 8:00 p.m. and he was "kicking ass." Before the evening hours at the model, he worked at his office and at the job sites starting every day before 7:00 a.m. He was always moving, always moving fast. He was tireless.

Summer vacations were rare because it was the frantic time for home building and farming. But when we did get away, unless it was the motorcycle trip we made every summer, he wanted to drag along every possible toy we had. "Let's bring the boat and we can put the four-wheeler in the back of my pick-up. You can pull the horse trailer and bring four horses and we'll do a pack trip too." More than once I had a hard time talking him out of these grand plans. There was never enough time in any day to do all he wanted to do. I'm not sure it ever occurred to him to say the word "can't."

Maggie

I first laid eyes on Rockey in October 1989, at the Homebuilder's annual award ceremony and banquet. It's a big night for builders and developers, with coveted awards for the best design, marketing materials and residential development in all price ranges. Picture a very large banquet room in a fancy downtown hotel with windows overlooking the Minneapolis skyline, filled with upwards of four hundred hardworking people from the construction industry, dressed in their best attempts to look successful, milling about meeting and greeting and shaking hands before the start of the main event.

My marketing company had a client list heavily represented by those in the room. My company was competing for awards in several categories. Like everyone else, I was dressed up that night and thought I looked pretty good. I was wearing a floaty black dress, my hair turned out, and I was very thin after a couple years of big personal losses. My mom died in May of 1987, followed by a divorce, the death of my dad and one of my dearest friends in less than two years. As I made my way through the crowd to say hello and wish good luck to clients, I scanned ahead looking for familiar faces. And there he was ... definitely not familiar.

He was taller than most in the room and when our eyes met, his smile was warm and a little more than electric. I felt him watching me as I made my way to his side of the room. As I moved through the crowd, I tried to resist the pull of this guy and began to veer away from his little knot of people. He took two long steps and stopped in my path. I looked up at his name tag—he was almost a foot taller than me—and said, "Oh jeez, you pretended to be out of business when I called last year. I was the coordinator for the Homes Section of the St. Paul Pioneer Press and called you for the town home section."

He smiled huge and said, "I lied."

I returned the smile and kept moving, wondering what the hell just happened. I had a physical and chemical reaction to him like no one before, ever. I was glad to reach my table and sit down, but soon realized that across the room, he had turned his chair some and was looking right at me with that big beard and bigger smile. My night was doomed. The dinner and award show were long but nice, and I won several prizes for big projects. I snuck a look at him more than once and found there was no sneaking. Each time my eyes met his, staring back at me with that great smile and big beard. That damn smile had some current in it. His company also took several design awards in three different price categories. When the show was over, I walked quickly to the elevators, wanting to beat the traffic. As I stepped into the elevator and pressed the down button a big hand shot in the door, and there was that smile standing above me once more. The smile said, "I can't let you go without knowing your name." Smiling stupidly, I told him my name and my company name, slipped a business card out of my pocket and into his hand and the doors slid shut.

It was years later that I realized that encounter was completely out of character for the shy, reserved guy with the winning smile.

In 1993, I moved to the farm in North Branch, Minnesota with Rockey and his teenage son Nick. The house and one barn were done. We finished fencing the front forty acres that fall and brought a herd of pregnant Scottish Highland cows home and split some pastures off for them and the horses. The fencing continued as soon as the snow melted, and a horse barn went up. I started breeding gaited horses, and by the next spring, the babies of cows and horses were all thriving under my care. Rockey bought more land and built a huge shop to work on big trucks and farm equipment. We built more fences and got more cattle, delivered calves and foals, bought more tractors and plowed, tilled, baled hay and planted our way into a pretty big farming outfit. We both worked full time and neither of us, both strong and fit, minded the never-ending farm work after long days at our real jobs. I grew up on a family farm in El Paso, Wisconsin, so the rhythms of wins and losses from weather and agriculture prices was natural to me. But for suburban kid Rockey, not so much. His force of nature way of getting things done was a key to many of his successes, but held little sway over a corn-killing hailstorm or a nine-inch rain on a newly sprouted alfalfa field. I remember the look on his face as he drove up one day to find me covered in mud and goo carrying a newborn calf away from its dead mother. I calmly looked up and said, "Get the tractor and loader out, will you? We need to get that mama out of here." He had no farm experience and mine was useless, except by example, to help him learn who was really in charge of bounty on the farm. He could roll with changes and adjust to accommodate obstacles on a construction site, but the whims of Mother Nature were beyond his ability to cope with. I secretly smiled sometimes at his stunned realization that he'd finally met something he couldn't control.

As the 1990s sped by, we both experienced successes and failures in our business lives. The farm continued to thrive and produce new life every year as a result of long hours, hard work and some luck. We clashed over methods on the crop portion of the farm and eventually divided the management of it into two distinct and separate parts. Rockey oversaw the crops and when Tim came over to help, he mostly worked with Rockey in the fields while I managed the livestock and breeding programs. It ended up being the best farm decision we made, even though it became one more way to allow us to avoid collaboration and maintain an odd separateness that defined our relationship.

There were more adventures. We continued to indulge our shared love of Big Sky in the winter and the Montana backcountry the rest of the year. A good member of the concrete crew, a guy named Doc, became our go-to person to watch over the farm and animals while we traveled. Doc was a city guy and loved these farm vacations. Even with no experience, he developed a keen eye for the health of both cows and horses, and I'm pretty sure he let the dogs sleep in bed with him. Every year we would buy a dozen or so feeder pigs and raise them through the summer. We sold most of them to our friends, but we kept one for ourselves, to be butchered in the fall.

The night before we left on one of our road trips, I would always make an inspection round of the animals, checking them for wellness. One night I noticed one of the pigs I'd been doctoring had died. I walked the half mile back up to the shop and found Rock and asked him to come and help me get the dead pig out of the area we called The Pig Palace. Night was falling and the September temperatures were cool, so we each got ahold of two legs and tossed the pig out of the Palace and dragged him about thirty feet away. We both had a ton of things to finish before our early morning departure and went back to loading the trailer and the truck. The pig was forgotten. I left a detailed note for Doc about the status of everything, and we loaded horses and hit the road by 6:00 a.m., heading for Montana. A couple days later, after a long day in the saddle to scout out a place for an elk camp in the high country, we fed the horses and returned to the condo to eat. Doc called to check in and ran through the list of good and bad on the farm. At the end of the conversation, Doc said in a secretive voice, "So yeah, about them pigs. Do they kill their own?" After some uproarious laughter from me, he told the story of finding the dead pig. Since I had neglected to tell him about it, he thought the pigs had done it. Good old Doc was greatly relieved to find out that no, they do not kill their own.

The farm was about a half hour north of the Twin Cities suburb of Lino Lakes, where Rockey's office and concrete company shop were located. My office was in a picturesque little river town of Stillwater on the border between Minnesota and Wisconsin, also about a half hour away. We moved in together shortly after Rockey's divorce was final. He and Tim had started both companies— the concrete company and the home building company—when they were in their early twenties. Those companies employed some family and long-term friends that were much like family. I was viewed as the interloper and mostly treated with open hostility, and I rarely went to his office or had much interaction with the office staff. The boys on the crews were not so inclined to be mean to me, and I was very comfortable stopping in to say hello at the job sites. Rockey's partner Tim was also pretty involved with the farm, and he and I enjoyed a solid friendship during the years of my life with Rockey. The biggest hardship was the hate and blame directed at me for Rockey's divorce. I didn't earn that, but it was easier for his ex-wife to call it that way than to admit their mul tiple separations indicated trouble long before he ever heard my name. His sons chose sides early. The older son, Rock Jr., chose to live with his mom and barely spoke to his father and never to me for many years. Nick lived with us and thrived there for a while. After we'd been at the farm for about two years, Nick started to see his mom again. She was accommodating to his seventeen-year-old brother and his friends to party and drink at their house, so it made sense, after one weekend visit, Nick opted to move back with her, quit school and spend his days drinking and partying. It was a bad place for a couple of kids with the predilection for bad decisions, and it broke Rockey's heart. If he blamed me for Nick's exodus, he never said so. The poison toward me escalated over the years, further alienating the boys from their father. Girlfriends of both boys seemed to enjoy telling me stories of drunken campfire talks with Rockey's ex-wife where hours were spent trashing me. It didn't matter that I owned my own business, made my own money, enjoyed my own success long before I met Rockey, and paid my own way. I was the gold-digging bitch who was out to rob their father. None of the stories told around those drunken campfires were true because none of them had ever asked me one single question about who I was or what I stood for. Much to my dismay, I don't believe that Rockey ever stood up for me. I am sure neither kid spoke harshly about me in front of Rockey, but the animosity story was told and retold in the tight circle that they lived within. For nearly thirty years, I believed that if Rockey had said just once, "I love her and she makes my life a better place," the volume on the hate machine would have been turned way down. He never did and it was a wedge between us that started tiny and only grew wider over the decades.

Stem Cells
2005

The year 2005 was all about getting settled in the house in Gallatin Gateway and finishing construction projects on the farm in Montana. We had intended to spend our time split between the farm in Minnesota and the new place, but it never worked out that way. Everything about being in Montana felt right. It felt as if I was finally home. I made a couple trips back to Minnesota and Rock came along on the first one in May. We packed clothes, housewares, tools and tack into my two-horse trailer. Rockey would drive the big trailer back to Montana full of horses and mules. Our intention was to stay in Minnesota for a few weeks, see some people and say some goodbyes, but upon arrival at the old farm, we instantly knew that it was no longer home. The pastures felt empty with the cattle gone, and the sale of all but forty acres had diminished the fun of it so significantly, we practically threw our belongings into the trailer. My need to be back in Montana was largely emotional. I knew it was where I wanted and needed to be. I had a gypsy heart and never felt much attachment to place. Montana changed that for me, and what I wanted most was to be home. For Rock, I think he was anticipating all the projects waiting for him at our new place: things to build, a shop to finish out, and all the building of things he loved to do. We never even took a last horse ride through the woods and the trails that Rock had made for us in Minnesota. I didn't call anyone, friends or family, as I tore through the house looking for important things to take, and Rockey only visited Tim once, and then we were turned around, headed back for Montana in less than a week.

So sure were we about where we needed to be, there were no goodbyes, no farewell parties, not even a slip of paper with our new address. It felt right and freeing to do it that way and neither of us second-guessed our getaway. Hauling six horses and mules, the best part was driving straight through the 1,041 miles from door to door, fifteen and a half hours caravanning as fast as we could drive. We arrived at our home in Gallatin Gateway just before dusk, unloaded the gang and stood by the fence smiling as they bucked and ran through their new pasture.

About half of the eighty acres that we bought in Gateway and reimagined into a farm had been an alfalfa field for decades. We hoped to make a deal with the neighbor, who had been cutting and baling it for the last owner, to do the same for us and split the hay as payment. We had sold all our haymaking implements and only brought a tractor and a Bobcat for farm work. The best thing about having someone else cut hay was not having to spend those long, hottest days of summer putting up hay. The very bad thing about it is the loss of any control over when the hay is cut. Rockey decided he had made enough hay in this lifetime, seemingly okay with the new arrangement, until he realized the hay wasn't going to get cut on the precise day he thought it had reached its zenith because the hay-cutting guy was cutting someone else's hay that day. As soon as the neighbor finished his work at our place, Rock, wearing his master of the universe cape, scoured Craigslist and drove all over this big state, buying a swather, a rake and two balers so he could reclaim his haymaking crown in the next season.

The amount of physical and mental stress on Rockey from building the new place started to become evident that summer. When he was diagnosed in 2002, Dr. Tuite told him that exhaustion from Parkinson's was inevitable and that Rock would benefit from daily naps, a suggestion that Rockey thought was probably a good idea for other people. In this summer three years later, he started taking those naps and his physical prowess showed the strain when he missed one. His tremor became more pronounced, the left foot drop more noticeable, and he was more uncoordinated in the late afternoon of the napless days. It was obvious to him that the benefit outweighed his pride, so an hour nap became part of most days. The difference in his physical ability was so apparent, I did my best to encourage naps, even lying down with him sometimes. That created a whole different benefit in Rockey's eyes, and although I tried not to make it a habit, the promise of a roll in the hay was a good nap enticement.

We still had much work to do that summer. I also had a crown to reclaim as landscaper/gardener extraordinaire. I hauled rocks, ran tillers, dragged, seeded and reseeded the yard and roped Rock into doing some fancy Bobcat work to add some earth and a huge stone structure for my landscaping projects. There were trees, shrubs, a perennial garden or three and a vegetable garden to plant in order to turn an alfalfa field into a homestead. Rockey was pressing his old skills as a concrete guy into service, pouring floors in the horse barn and the shop and adding slabs outside each building. Finishing concrete is brutal work. It requires long concrete rakes, kneepads, trowels and speed. It was outrageously taxing for an aging concrete man and a short-armed woman. He poured a big slab next to the horse barn with electric, septic and water hookups for an RV, so Tim could visit anytime. We built a tack room in the horse barn and work benches in the big shop. It was an endless list of projects that we mostly had wrapped up by the time the archery elk season opened around Labor Day.

The work of setting up the high-country camp with the wall tent seemed like a day at the county fair after the summer of strong arms and aching backs. Rockey would stay up there for weeks at a time that fall with visiting hunter friends, coming out every ten days to resupply food and beer. I stayed only a couple of nights in camp to help set up, riding down the mountain with a smile on my face, proud that I hadn't gotten talked into being the camp cook for a bunch of smelly boys wearing camo. Fall was a rejuvenating time for both of us. With Rock in camp, I started exploring trailheads in the canyon, seeking places to hike, ride horse and explore on my own. I hiked and rode horse for miles that fall, not realizing I was discovering wild places I would come to rely on to reclaim my peace in the coming years. The solitude felt luxurious after a year of constant motion and the voices of workers.

We flew back to Minneapolis for Christmas in 2005. Rockey's family held a Christmas Eve dinner at his sister's stately home in old St. Paul. It was unspoken, but nonetheless a command performance for everyone in the family. Janet, Rock's mom, who was dancing on the edge of Alzheimer's, was always the best part of the evening. She was kind, funny and easy to love. It mattered to her that she got everyone in one place on this one day, so we all showed up. Two full years after his diagnosis, Rockey still hadn't told anyone in his immediate family about his Parkinson's disease. His reason for not telling his mom was simple: he didn't want her to worry. He became skilled at hiding his worsening left-hand tremor by touching something or the pocket trick he used early on. He had discovered that if he reached for something with his left hand, say a saltshaker, the tremor stopped—hence the name resting tremor. This understanding allowed him to quiet the shaking, temporarily anyway, by either using that hand or by twirling a small stone in his pocket. Rock was pleased when another year of family holiday gathering passed, and no one seemed to notice.

We were staying with my childhood friend Tracy, who had a beautiful home on the St. Croix River, the Scenic Waterway that separates Minnesota and Wisconsin. My family in Wisconsin hadn't had a Christmas gathering for years, so Tracy and her daughter Tessa and I had been holding our own special holiday celebrations. Ours were laid back with good food, much laughter, perfectly chosen gifts and lots of love around.

Later in the celebration evening, Tracy started a conversation about her brother-in-law and his brothers in California working with stem cells on patients with neurological issues. They seemed to have had some success treating stroke patients and several spinal cord injuries. There were four brothers, all with one or more doctorate degrees. Only one—I'll call him Jay—was a medical doctor as well as having advanced degrees in nutrition and homeopathic medicine. They employed several Russian scientists at their California lab, and they were doing the research as well as growing and developing the stem cells. Tracy believed they might be interested in treating Rockey, and she agreed to make a phone call to lay some groundwork and get some contact information. Rockey was very interested in this development as there were no options available in traditional Western medicine for treating Parkinson's other than the increasing dosages of drug cocktails.

The drugs used to treat PD are effective at minimizing the more obvious physical symptoms. At the time, there were five main drugs prescribed to Parkinson's patients. Rockey took a very low dose of Mirapex. It helped to quiet the tremors, but he mainly relied on it to stop the leg spasms at night. Typically, the neurologists will start a patient on a drug to relieve one or more of the symptoms. Most, if not all, of these drugs have a short window of efficacy, so after an average of three years, they begin to cocktail the drugs. This means that the patient continues to take the original drug with its waning effects but adds another to smooth out and boost the effectiveness, therefore lengthening the hours of the day that symptoms are relieved. There is a particular drug called Sinemet that is the end-game drug. The idea being that the patient would use all the other drugs in various combinations, saving Sinemet for last, as it is seen as the best one. It also has the shortest window of effectiveness and terrible side effects. I was still doing the research he needed to make informed medical decisions. My findings on

Sinemet prompted Rockey to say he would never take that drug because the side effects were so debilitating. My thoughts were the same as they were in the beginning—his disease, his body, his decisions—so when I presented the knowledge I had gained through research, I tried to keep my opinions to myself unless he asked.

As he looked down the road, all Rock could see was being a slave to an ever-increasing cocktail of drugs that would make him slow, stupid and uncoordinated. He seemed particularly sensitive to drugs at this stage of his life, and he was loath to consider increasing doses, which did nothing to slow the progression, but just masked symptoms. His doctor tried to convince him to add another drug to help with the increasing rigidity in one leg, and even though he had picked up the prescription, he was resistant to it. He was excited to investigate the prospect of stem cell treatment.

After we returned to Montana, Tracy got me the contact information for the stem cell brothers. I called, left messages and finally connected with her brother-in-law, Monty, and gave him Rockey's current condition, agreeing to send his medical records. Then there was a four-month silence until Jay called and said they would like to include Rock in their stem cell transplant program. Rockey had several conversations with Jay and one of the scientists while they explained the procedure. They sent a very extensive contract and non-disclosure agreement with plenty of language about proprietary information, experimental treatments, no guarantees and possible side effects. We learned that the airline tickets to Russia were $5,900 each, the hotel would be around $3,000 and the treatment itself would cost $25,000—a cashier's check prior to departure, please. This was happening at a time when Rockey had the most personal wealth and ability to turn it into cash. We had sold nearly everything when we made the Montana move. His practice of frugality was tossed when he made the decision to pursue the stem cell treatments, and he never regretted that decision. This was during the George W. Bush years and Bush's ban on embryonic stem cell research in the US, to please the Evangelicals, had been called out by the Parkinson's Disease Foundation and particularly by Michael J. Fox, whose foundation had been raising millions for Parkinson's research. It was during the stem cell ban that Rush Limbaugh, with cameras rolling, callously mocked Michael J. Fox and his tremors. This ban in the United States was the reason the stem cell brothers had formed a collaboration with the leading Parkinson's doctor in Russia and the Russian government. Turns out, the Russians had been using stem cells to treat neurological issues for thirty years, a total smack to my American arrogance.

We were given a contact named Ellie from a travel agency in San Diego, and I made arrangements to fly to Moscow in early November. Obtaining visas and other permissions in two months' time was difficult, but Ellie was a seasoned international travel agent and somehow made all the meetings at the consulate work so it all came together. She later said that trying to get the package of travel documents overnighted to Montana was the biggest hurdle of all; I laughed and told her overnight delivery was just a dream in our state as I drove 85 mph to the Butte Post Office and back to retrieve the documents just hours before our plane took off. We flew to LA and stayed close to the airport. I got a map and looked for something to do, then called a cab that drove us to Venice Beach in the early evening hours. I loved all the weirdness and the colorful people. Rockey and I walked around, avoided talking about Russia, ate some street food and laughed at ourselves feeling so out of place in this world of buff bodies, tiny clothes and very good sunglasses. It all looked so lighthearted and at least superficially happy while we grappled with the weight of a looming and risky procedure, with no guarantees, in a dangerous part of the world.

We met up with two of the stem cell brothers at LAX and went through the lines and check-in rigamarole. We boarded an Aeroflot direct flight to Moscow, took our seats in business class and belted in for the fifteen-hour flight. The plane was more modern than anything I'd been exposed to. Each passenger in our part of the plane had their own pod-looking seat. The seat was fabulously comfortable, a little bit like a chair caress, and moved into thirty-five different positions, which turned out to be a necessity on a flight that long. Many of the passengers were regulars on this flight and disappeared into the restrooms only to emerge in baggy sweats and slippers to offset the bad ways a body swells up on a very long flight. We didn't know. We sat there with our too-tight jeans and laced up shoes, wishing we weren't such hicks.

Our high anxiety wasn't only about the treatment itself but was also made significantly more intense by being in Russia. We had paid extra for VIP Customs at Sheremetyevo International Airport at the suggestion of the stem cell brothers, but even with that it was an intimidating process. Taken to a basement room, we were escorted into a beautiful space with dark paneling and an elegant bar with plush seating at small tables scattered about. The chairs were filled with mostly well-dressed men and I heard not a word of English. Rockey and I stuck close to the stem cell brothers, falling short of hanging onto their coats. An announcement blared, and Jay said, "This is us," and they took us down a dark, low-ceilinged hallway to another room nothing like the fancy bar. They examined documents and passports then stamped them, the customs agent asking us questions in Russian that someone in our group answered. Moments later, we got into a red Aerostar minivan with a guy named Alex, who drove us to a ritzy American chain hotel near Red Square. After taking our bags to our room, we met the stem cell brothers in the hotel bar and they finally spoke some truths. There was another, bigger man at the table whose name was also Alex. He was to be my minder for the duration of our stay. Since Rockey would be in the hospital for most days, I was to stay in Alex's company at all times. If I wasn't in my hotel room, I was to be with Alex.

"Alex will take you wherever you need to go," they told me. "He will take you to the hospital and wait for you for as long as you wish to stay." The area around the hotel looked like an upscale urban area and safe, so I asked if I could go for walks. "Alex will take you wherever you want to go," was the answer.

"Rockey will be with one of us at all times," a brother said.

"Can I go over to the little bodega across the street?" I asked. Rockey kicked me under the table.

"Alex will take you to the bodega," I was told.

Once I let go of my quest to be on my own, the conversation grew serious, and they revealed more details of the treatment. To-morrow, on his first day in the hospital, Rockey would undergo a pre-surgery check-up and a more involved assessment performed by Dr. M., the immensely qualified Parkinson's specialist in Russia and other parts of the world, who would actually be the person ad-ministering the stem cell transplant. The brothers told us in mostly lay terms that the transplant would take place two or three days from now. They would sedate Rockey with light anesthesia while the doctor performed a lumbar puncture, commonly referred to as a spinal tap. The doctor would then, using a large bore needle, remove what looked to be a couple teaspoons of spinal fluid. They would then inject an equal amount of stem cell solution, which was hundreds of millions of this kind of cell and that kind of cell (I am not allowed to be specific) suspended in a liquid compatible to his own spinal fluid, into Rockey's spinal column to replace the fluid just removed. He needed to stay in bed for twenty-four hours, totally flat, no moving, a common precaution after a lumbar puncture. At this early chapter in American stem cell research, the belief was that the cells injected into the spine would migrate to the brain and work to fix or mend the damaged parts of Rock's brain—specifically, the substantia nigra where dopamine is pro-duced. These were not brain-specific stem cells, but rather a type of cell used to adapt to any damaged part of the human body. After the procedure, Rockey would be under doctor supervision for the full twenty-four hours and would remain in the hospital for a few days. They gave Rockey and me cell phones with all the players' numbers pre-programmed and told us to never even turn on our own phones. They also told us that if we were questioned by any-one, we were to say we were tourists seeing the sights in Moscow. As the medical talk wound down, Jay asked about our Minnesota life. We talked jobs, the farm and of course horses. Jay told us he had been a roommate of a good friend of ours, ridden horses with another couple we knew well and been a close friend with our veterinarian. Small world. It became clear to both Rock and me that Jay was the brother we felt most comfortable with, and as the years went by, we grew to consider him a friend. Luckily for us and particularly Rockey, Jay was our main contact for the six-year relationship with the stem cell company. Of all the people we met and dealt with during the stem cell chapter, Jay was the one who answered every question, returned every phone call and made sure Rockey was well taken care of in this complicated process.

We slept well in our beautiful hotel room and met the brothers and others in the dining room for breakfast. After we ate, we loaded into two vans and headed across Moscow for the hospital with Alex, my minder, in the driver's seat. It was November with a chill in the air similar to our weather in Montana. What I remember most was the gray. The sky was gray, every building we passed was gray, the pedestrians faces were gray. After a few minutes of travel, I asked where all the houses were and what were all those huge gray buildings. Alex told me that houses are rare, only for the very rich and in another part of the city, and that those gray buildings were apartment buildings. He said that most Muscovites live in similar buildings, and the apartments were very, very small. Alex had been educated in America, and he gave a little chuckle with an eyebrow wag when he told me, "Small by American standards." I remember thinking I would have so many questions for Alex as the days went by. When we pulled up to the hospital, it looked modern and well-kept. A landscaped circular drive had an array of flags with the Russian flag flying highest. The seven of us entered through a side door and went directly to what would be Rockey's room. That initial impression was the only thing that looked modern and well kept. The building was ancient with linoleum that looked like a 1960s vintage, a little bit sticky and certainly dull.

Rockey's room was large and on the ground floor with big windows that opened. It had plastic curtains, a small twin bed, one hard-backed chair and a private bathroom, which smelled strongly of urine and had stains to accompany the smell. I felt a little guilty when I pictured my luxurious room at the fancy hotel with a wonderful bed, clean bathroom with a double shower, cable TV and killer breakfast with excellent coffee. I stood off to the side while everyone talked to Rockey and helped make him comfortable. Soon, more doctors came into the room, and we were introduced to the famous Russian neurologist and his son, who shared their practice, as well as Raffi, a visiting neurologist from Armenia who had done a residency in California and had been working with the stem cell brothers for about a year. They were all charming and welcoming. The three Russian doctors then whisked Rock away for a day of testing and exams and I left with Alex with a plan to return later in the day. He was kind enough to take me on a driving tour of important sites in Moscow, and I found him to be quite dry but entertaining and surprisingly free with answers to my questions. I asked how he got hooked up with these guys, and he said he had done some cellular research for them when he had finished up one of his PhD programs. He told me he had two PhDs—one in Cellular Biology and another in Physics. He worked for the Russian government doing research, getting paid an equivalent of $200 a month, while working parttime for the stem cell brothers for occasional patient spouses, getting paid $800 per month. His English was excellent, one of the reasons he had gotten the job. It was dangerous for a non-Russian speaking American to be on their own, so the stem cell company felt it lessened their liability enough to warrant having a person like Alex to watch over people like me. Once I was in my room, I was to call Alex if I wanted to go anywhere outside of the hotel. When I did, he was always waiting for me when I got off the elevator. I appreciated it, but the presence of Alex created some anxiety too, wondering what would happen to me if Alex wasn't there.

He took me back to the hospital around 4:00 p.m. that day and I walked in Rock's room only to be followed in by the Russian big doctor and his son. They propped themselves on the wide windowsills and just hung out and visited with us. The older of the two knew where Montana was and was aware of its beauty. He noticed a pack of Kool cigarettes sticking out of Rockey's bag and asked if he could have one. Rock said sure and the son asked if we had any non-menthols. I ponied up my Winston Lights and both doctors were beaming, declaring their love for American cigarettes. Then to our shock, each of them cranked open a window and lit up, chain smoking and smiling with their new best friends, laughing about how uptight Americans are. At some point in the smoke-a-thon, a woman showed up with a tray of Rock's dinner. Everyone cleared out and I set his dinner tray on a little table and removed the metal cover, making no comment. Rock stared at it for a minute and looked at me with wide eyes and asked what I thought it was.

"It's boiled tongue and boiled potatoes," I said.

He said, "Well it smells like feet and I'm not touching it … please get it away from me."

I was cracking up as I carefully sealed in the stink with the cover and set the dish on the floor by the door. I had packed lots of crackers and peanut butter and some other food, so I dug that out and made Rockey a plate, vowing to find some take-out for him tomorrow. The woman who brought the food came back, lifted the cover and started to chatter at Rockey in Russian. He puffed his belly out and pointed at the debris from his cracker-and-peanut-butter meal and tried to signal that he was full. She gestured at him with the covered tongue and said more, becoming quite excited walking toward us brandishing the plate. Finally, Rock stopped patting his puffed-out belly and said forcefully "Nyet! Nyet!" The poor lady turned and walked away, seemingly sad at her lack of success with the important American patient.

There was no cable TV at the hospital, but I had brought a tiny-screened DVD player and a stack of movies. I set him up with The Godfather, gave him a kiss and got back into the Aerostar with Alex to head back to the hotel for the night. I did not feel guilty ordering a room service pot of coffee and a fruit plate when I settled in. I did have cable TV, but the only English-speaking shows were CNN London and Meerkats on the Animal Planet. For the next few days, I saw endless coverage of Tom Cruise and Katie Holmes' wedding and every Meerkats show ever produced. The whole idea of watching that obsessive wedding coverage in a nice hotel in Moscow was but one of the weird things about being there, and I was grateful to have brought so many books.

I stayed at the hotel the next morning, and Rock called me around 9:00 a.m. He was whispering in the phone that they were taking him to the basement, and he was worried that if the rooms were this awful, what could possibly be in the basement? He wanted me to know where he was going in case they never brought him back. I told him it was probably full of the most cutting-edge medical equipment and not to worry. Later, he told me it was indeed super clean and modern, like stepping into another world. They finished with the scans and testing by noon, so Alex took me to the hospital. This time when they brought food, there were several dishes on the tray and Rock smiled and nodded at the lady who brought them. Under the cover was a piece of boiled fish, unrecognizable except for the smell, and a big pile of boiled potatoes. A smaller cover revealed a pink soup that I knew immediately and smiled. Rockey had a laughable disdain for beets, one of my favorite foods, and I had often teased him about it. He smelled it and stared at it for a moment and looked up at me and asked what I thought it was.

"Borsht," I said. "It's a kind of soup."

He looked at it some more and said, "What do they use to make pink soup?"

I guffawed and said, "It's delicious, it's beets!"

After slamming the cover back on, he decided that potatoes would be good and had a pack of Nutter Butter cookies for dessert, asking me to please bring him some better food. I called Jay and asked how I could go about getting some food for Rock and he said, "I got it, don't worry." The next night and for the rest of his hospital stay, Jay showed up every day with terrific take-out food. They would administer the stem cells the next day around noon.

The Russian doctors prepped and performed the procedure right in Rockey's room. Although I was invited to watch, I declined. I stayed while they explained it again and gave Rockey some anesthesia. I met the English-speaking nurse named Olga they had hired to stay with Rockey for the whole twenty-four hours. Another very friendly person, Olga was a substantial woman at close to six feet tall, heavily made-up and sporting gigantic eyebrows. Bathing in Russia was only an occasional practice, which they attempted to compensate for by wearing large amounts of potent perfume or cologne. While I visited with Olga in the hallway during the procedure, I tried to remember to breathe through my mouth and not stare at those eyebrows sitting atop the bluest eyeshadow I'd ever seen. It didn't take long before I was called back in. Rock was groggy and slept most of the afternoon. We shared a takeout dinner and Alex took me back to the hotel.

At close to midnight, my phone rang, and it was Jay. They had all been out to dinner when Jay got a call that Rockey was in distress. Raffi was on call at the hospital and tending to him. He had spiked a fever of 103°F, his heart rate was elevated, and he was delirious. Jay was rushing to the hospital, and they didn't want me to come. I muted the Meerkats and broke down and cried. The difficulty of the language barriers and the lack of control over everything crashed in on me. I was so worried and had never experienced not being able to be by his side for a medical emergency. I knew he would be terrified. I paced and cried and ordered more coffee, waiting to hear something, when finally, around 2:00 a.m., Jay called and said they had gotten his fever and his heart rate down, but they had to administer some heavy sedation in order to accomplish that. I asked if Olga would be the only one there for the rest of the night, and I was told that she had gotten so drunk, she passed out on the couch in his room and that was how his vitals became so extreme because she hadn't been checking on him.

So, Dr. Raffi would stay in his room and monitor him to avoid any further crisis. I didn't sleep much and rode with Alex back to hospital first thing in the morning. Rock was heavily sedated and would remain so throughout the day, so I was taken back to hotel where I slept like the dead until the next morning.

I had never really wanted to go to Moscow but couldn't abide the idea of Rockey not having me there for back-up. He was so optimistic about this experimental treatment that I couldn't live with myself not giving it my best effort to be supportive. But when I finally awoke and was getting ready to go back to hospital, I found a new dislike and fear of the whole Russian adventure. They had no concrete explanations for Rock's extreme reaction to the stem cells and they decided to keep him sedated to ensure his heart rate didn't go crazy again. He slept most of that day, and I just wedged into the tiny bed and curled up behind him while he slept. I stayed in the room with him that night, ate Nutter Butter cookies with bad coffee, and watched him sleep and visited every so often with Raffi when he came to check on Rockey. They weaned him off the sedation, and his vitals all stayed normal, so he was released mid-afternoon and we went back to the hotel, where he slept until morning. That day, Alex picked us up and took us on a tour. We saw the old KGB building, which was now home to the FSK, the intelligence agency that replaced the KGB, although Alex told us that a new name did not mean their practices were any more humane. We walked around Red Square and toured a famous cathedral and saw all the sights that we Americans recognize as iconic Russian architecture. In the early afternoon, I asked Rock how he was feeling, and he said not so good. He was so dopey he couldn't remember where we had been for the past couple of hours, so I asked Alex to take us back. Once again, he slept the rest of the day, and we went to dinner that night with other patients from around the world who were there for stem cell treatments as well. The food was fabulous, and we met some people we would stay in touch with for many years. Rockey remembered nothing about that evening. We boarded the flight home and when we returned to LAX it looked like heaven to me.

Dirty Earl, a Grizzly Bear and Brain Surgery

2006-2010

By January of 2007, there was a full-time tenant living with the uneasy task of getting rid of the mice that had taken over the North Branch farm in our absence. Rockey listed the Minnesota farm for sale, and we had settled into an easy rhythm in Montana. Rockey had agreed to supervise a project in Big Sky for a friend named Jeff, who wanted to build a commercial building. Over the winter, he and Jeff worked on plans and started the bidding process for the subcontractor pieces of the job.

In March, Rock and I went to Billings to the Outfitters Horse and Mule Sale. We were hoping to find a replacement for one of our aging pack mules. There were a couple of outfitters who we knew well enough to consult about some of the mules we spotted. We drove home that day with Dirty Earl in the trailer. He was a handsome fella, about fifteen hands tall (a hand is four inches and the term is used to measure the height of horses and mules at the withers), charcoal gray with four white stockings. He came from a reputable outfitter in Wyoming who had been using Earl for packing and carrying dudes on trail rides. We set him up in a quarantine pen and slowly, over the next few weeks, introduced him to our herd. Our mules were funny about newcomers to their herd because they didn't care at all. The horses had to do a little neck-arched prancing with some kicks and bucks thrown in just for fun, but they didn't make much trouble for Earl either.

On a sunny Sunday afternoon in early April, Rock decided to take Dirty Earl for a spin. He seemed perfectly calm and well-mannered as Rock tacked him up. I got my horse Tommy ready to go and we were in the lead so Earl could follow a quiet horse and get his bearings. As we rounded a corner in the alfalfa field, maybe a half mile into the ride, Rock was happy and said what a nice, smooth ride Earl was, and he was going to take the lead for a while. Things were going perfectly for the next mile or so and we walked slowly around the field, and then suddenly Earl was in the air. He did one big leap and took a hard left and started to buck over and over, higher than a rodeo bronc. I watched Rockey trying to hang on until he finally decided to bail, while Earl's ass end was as high in the air as it could go. Rockey flipped end over end and landed with a thud. Dirty Earl took off at fast gallop heading for anywhere but here, and by then Tommy had managed to catch some adrenaline and was crow hopping his giant body, fighting against my wishes to go to where Rockey lay on the muddy spring ground. I got Tommy to stop dancing long enough to jump off to help Rock before Tommy tore off after Dirty Earl.

Rock was lying with his arms wrapped around his torso and clearly in pain. I offered to run and get the truck and he thought he could walk back the half mile to the house. I put my hand out for Rock to grab and he got to his feet, took two steps and fell back to the ground with a huge cry of pain, gasping for breath. He cried out, "I think my back is broken." I took off running and came bouncing back through the field driving my SUV. It was a struggle for tall Rockey to bend enough to get in, but he finally did, and I drove slowly to avoid tossing him around. Both Tommy and Earl had run right back to the barn, so I stopped and jumped out, took off the saddles and bridles, threw them on the ground and opened the gate for the boys to go back to the pasture. I continued to drive slowly down our long driveway and the gravel road out but punched the gas when I hit the highway.

The hospital was about a half hour away and we made it in less. I dashed in to get Rockey a wheelchair. He was pale, and his breathing was shallow and rapid. They admitted him to the E.R. and I sat in a blue hospital chair in Rockey's cubicle while we waited for a doctor. X-rays showed he had at least nine broken ribs, several shattered into small pieces, and the rest was undetermined because all the damage was on the curve of the ribs which didn't show up clearly on the imaging. They gave him a prescription for some pain meds and sent him home, saying they didn't even bandage broken ribs anymore and that he might want to sleep in a recliner for a few nights. I got him back into the house, removed his boots, stripped off his filthy, muddy jeans, slipped on some sweatpants and tried to help him get comfortable in the chair. The pain meds took the edge off, but he was far from comfortable. I slept on the couch nearby in case he needed help in the night.

By mid-morning the next day, his breathing had become even more labored, and his chest had a loud rattle, so I insisted that he get back to the hospital. Rock was pretty sure that he couldn't get back into the truck, to which I replied that the EMTs could carry him on a stretcher. God forbid the neighbors would see an ambulance come to our house, so he decided to get himself into the truck. After shuffling down some long hallways and waiting in the blue chairs, we finally saw his primary physician, who was so alarmed he had Rockey admitted to ICU in less than an hour. I felt relieved when a substantial team took him from me as I trailed behind them down some long hallways to the ICU. Once he was settled and they had administered morphine, they suggested I leave for a few hours as they tried to determine what was happening. This time they would use better imaging tools. I hurried back home, did the chores, let the dogs out, showered and drove back to the hospital just in time to catch a doctor coming out of his room. He confirmed the nine broken ribs and had also discovered a bruised lung and a bruised spleen. His main concern was getting Rockey's pain under control because the shallow breathing had caused fluid to build up in his lungs, causing pneumonia on both sides. As I walked through the curtain, I found a very pale Rockey, hooked up to oxygen, IV fluid, antibiotics and a morphine drip, sitting up in his bed. His face told me he was still in serious pain, but his voice said he was high as kite. He spoke slowly with less agitation than earlier and asked a nonsensical question with heavy-lidded eyes that wanted to close. I stayed awhile and eventually went home for the night with no updates on his condition or plan for his treatment.

His condition was worse when I arrived the next morning, and a nurse told me an anesthesiologist was coming to insert an epidural line in his back, directly above the shattered ribs, so Rockey could administer morphine directly with a little button. Later, that doctor arrived and ordered me and a nurse to sit Rockey up on the edge of the bed. The anesthesiologist plopped down on the end of the bed and started to read what looked like instructions for the device he was about to implant in Rockey, with the patient in excruciating pain. Moments ticked by, Rockey gasping for breath and the dopey doctor still reading.

I asked the nurse to help me lay Rock back down and took the doctor by the arm and led him into the hallway, where I proceeded to tear into him for his lack of awareness for his patient and his unprofessionalism for reading the how-to manual while his patient moaned. He finally got the thing placed and gave Rock an extra level of pain relief until he was totally gorked out. His speech was mushy, and he would nod off in the middle of a sentence; it was a welcome reprieve from seeing him in so much pain. Over the next few days, he had a respiratory therapist and several other doctors working on his case.

No one ever explained his condition or what the plan was, and he remained in a deeply drugged state, waking occasionally to talk

nonsense. At one point, a doctor said they wanted to insert a needle into his lung to check the fluid; they were worried about a dark
spot being blood in his lung. I quickly called my friend Tracy in
the Twin Cities who was an anesthetist, to get her opinion. She
said to avoid puncturing the lung at all costs because it carried a
high risk of infection. It was another opportunity to hone my skills
as Rockey's medical advocate, as I told the doctor that no way
would they be performing this risky procedure just to have a look-
see. That dark spot on the X-ray disappeared in the next two days,
and they released Rockey. Not once, in the eight days in ICU, did
they tell me that he was in mortal danger or even what his greatest
injuries were. He slept in that recliner for four months, and he
never regained his ability to take a deep breath. His rib cage was
twisted when it healed, so his sternum was no longer the center
of his chest. We walked out of that hospital with Rockey trying
to recover from what would be life-altering injuries, with no clear
diagnosis of what had been damaged and even less idea of how he
would come back from this.

The lessons I learned from that experience helped me to become
a vocal and adamant advocate for Rockey for the next thirteen
years, never letting a doctor skate away again without telling me
exactly what was happening and what they were doing to fix it.
When Rock was home and recuperating, I called the man from
Wyoming who had previously owned Dirty Earl. I told him the
whole story and ended by saying that he didn't owe me a thing, but
would he consider taking the mule back. He was incredibly kind
and responded by telling me that whenever I was ready to make
the trip, I could bring Earl back to him for a full refund.

By the time summer arrived, Rockey was able to drive his truck,
and he spent that summer overseeing the construction of a commercial building in Big Sky. He didn't have to perform physical
labor on that project, so he was able to supervise with no problems.
He set up the high camp that fall, and the motion of riding plus
the lifting and twisting to set up the camp took a toll. I'm sure
sleeping on a cot did his broken body no good. Rock had a lev-

el-headed, big mule named Pete who had been his main ride for several years. There were a couple of local guys who visited him that year to archery hunt out of his camp. They had good luck and arched a big bull elk. The kill wasn't too far from the camp, and Rockey was specific about the need to haul the gut pile away as they worked on cutting up the big animal. Since they were deep in bear country and there was plenty of daylight left, Rockey decided to pack out as much of the meat as he could. He loaded Berta with the elk, saddled Pete, mounted and turned to his pals and said, "Now remember to put the head, the cape and the shoulders high up in a tree," then he turned Pete and they headed down the mountain.

When he reached the trailhead, he texted a friend to retrieve the meat and settled in to wait. Darkness was gaining on Rockey, so he didn't waste any time turning around to return to camp once he loaded the meat into the pickup. About halfway up, the sky turned black, and the wind screamed when the clouds opened up and dumped rain, making the trail a slimy mess. But Rock never worried about a challenge, and he kept Pete pointed up the mountain until the hail started. They stopped under a tree and waited for it to let up, but by now the trail was running with rainwater and hailstones. Mules are about the most sure-footed critters a rider can ask for, and when Pete slipped and fell to his knees the second time, Rock knew he had to turn back. Down the mountain and back to the trailhead, he loaded up the two mules in the trailer and headed for our house down the canyon, about forty-five minutes away. He called on the way, and I was waiting at the barn when he pulled in about ten at night. I could see he was struggling with the pain of all that travel, so I got both mules untacked and put away and fixed a quick something for him to eat.

He crashed fast and hard, only to rise at dawn, tack up, load up and head back up the canyon for the long ride to the camp. Good old Peter was a sure and steady mule. He had never lost his head or been difficult in any way. When they got within a hundred yards of camp, Pete suddenly snorted and hopped a little sideways. His

long ears were on full alert as he came to a full stop, Berta snorted and danced behind, making Rockey scan the trees in front of
them. The shadows in the trees made it hard to pick out details,
so he pulled up his binoculars for a better view. There in the trees,
between Rock and the camp, was a huge cache covered in leaves
and dirt and looking very fresh, with antlers and one hoof of a big
bull elk sticking out the top. When Pete snorted again and tried to
turn away, Rockey caught the movement of a big boar grizzly sitting not far from the prize he guarded. That was enough for good
old Pete, and he whirled around and made fast tracks down the
trail dragging Berta behind, with Rockey hanging on for dear life.
Rock was able to rein Pete in and slow him down to a walk and
turn around again, knowing they would need to take a long detour
around the bear and his cache to get back to camp. The cause of the
bear problem was that the boys didn't tie the remaining elk high
enough in the tree. Fifteen feet up, it was more of a dinner bell
than a safety measure. One of the guys told me later that Rockey
was so mad at them that his face was crimson with veins bulging
out in his neck as he hollered about their carelessness. Since the
bear then took up residence not far from camp, hoping for another
meal, the elk season was finished for the high-country camp.

After he packed out as much of the camp as he could get on his
own, Rockey decided to finish out the archery season at our farm
in the Gallatin Valley. One of the reasons we lived where we did
was the resident elk herd of about 160 who liked to graze and
lounge about in our hayfields. They spent their summers in the
mountains above us, and as the seasons changed, they moved down
the mountain right onto our place. We were short on trees or any
kind of natural blind, so Rock built two small hunting shacks on
either end of our hayfield, cleverly placed to be close to the elk no
matter which way they were travelling. If he wasn't camping in the
high camp, this was a fine spot to arch an elk. That meant instead
of being gone for most of the seven-week archery season, he was
home. Having him home in the archery season did impact my ear-

ly fall way of life. I liked spending September and October riding my Good Yellow Horse Lenny four or five days a week. I had a fine friend named Karen who lived just across the valley. I could load up my pony and dogs and be over there in fifteen minutes. She had a sweet deal living on a huge ranch that had been sold to developers as a high-end housing development with large acreages for sale. When Karen lived there, most of the lots hadn't sold, so she lived in a 3,000-acre gated community of one house. Karen on her little black horse and me on the Good Yellow could ride for hours and never see any other people or cars. We could ride a different trail every time we went out. Although Rockey being home didn't stop the riding completely, he had begun calling me often when I was gone. I never knew for sure if he was worried about me or thinking I was off somewhere else, but the calls came more frequently and with them came a subtle but nagging pressure to cut my fun short and return home.

Mostly our relationship was on solid footing in those years, and Rockey liked to talk about his big ideas for new projects either on the farm or somewhere else. Based on what they saw of us, because we exuded that close-couple vibe, most of our friends would have thought we had long talks about deep subjects, but that wasn't true at all. Rockey talked about things he was going to do, and I listened and asked questions. Even though most talk was about himself, it was still interesting if for no other reason than to keep track of whatever the hell he was cooking up.

One night after dinner, we were sitting on the porch in the dark and he was bugling to call in the bulls. It didn't take long until three or four bulls came snorting, chuckling and grunting their response to the calls. It never quit being a thrill to hear them come in so close in the dark; we could hear them snapping off grass as they grazed. I was a pretty good cow caller and together we coaxed the elk into a wild symphony with their rut sounds, the whole herd eating, pushing, fighting, bugling and peeping as they surrounded the house. We'd sometimes sit out there in the dark having whispered conversations as we listened to them. It was always a comfortable time for Rockey to impart important information to me, maybe because our faces were hidden from each other or maybe just because it was such uncluttered time spent together. He quietly whispered, "I think I'm done with Pete. I think I'm done with riding mules." I asked what he meant, and he proceeded to tell me about the trips up and down to the camp, the big bear scare and Pete's sudden turn and run. He said, "I was so scared by the time I got him under control, I could only think of that horrible wreck last spring. It was all I could do to get back on him to get out of the mountains. I think I can't ride him anymore and you should help me find a good horse. I mean, you always ride a good horse, can't you find one for me?" I was so surprised I didn't answer right away. Rockey had gotten into mules because he thought they were the ultimate rough country ride. They don't get tired, their feet are like iron, and their gait is smooth while carrying a person through unbelievably rough ground. If you get a good one, they are usually unflappable and super smart. Pete was all that, and Rockey had been riding him for years. He relied on Pete as a traveling partner, had trusted him over some really rough ground and took great pride in riding this big, beautiful black mule. I was stunned.

In my silence he finished his thoughts, "If I have another wreck like that one, I'll never walk again. I'm still not healed, Parkinson's makes everything worse, and I'll never be totally right again. The Parkinson's is messing with my balance, and I just don't feel that safe on Pete anymore. I've never been scared before, but when he saw that bear and turned around, I couldn't stop him, and it scared me too bad to ever do that again." That was an enormous admission for Rockey. I thought about how monumental it must have been in his mind, first to actually be physically scared, to recognize these losses and then to say it out loud. I assured him I could find him a steady-eddy good strong horse and that I'd start looking right away. Rock said, "Thanks. Make sure he's really handsome too, okay?" Thus ended the era of the riding mules and the start of the giving things up era.

In November, Rockey boarded another flight to Moscow to receive his second stem cell treatment. I didn't go this time, so he traveled with Jay, never telling him about the mule wreck or the injuries he suffered. It was an uneventful trip with no adverse reaction to the stem cells. Jay had a long talk with Rockey about how they perceived the stem cells working and his words served me well over the years as I tried to explain Parkinson's to people along the way. He said, "Think of Parkinson's as an evil Pac-Man in your brain. It never stops and moves slowly through, destroying brain cells. It is our hope that the stem cells will act as a wall in front of the Pac-Man, not curing your disease, but with a little luck, slowing down the destruction." We were always reminded that this treatment was experimental. The awareness of his silent nemesis was never far from my thoughts as we lived our life, moving through our world with many parts of Rock's physicality still intact. He kept up with that original promise to live faster and bigger while he had time, leaving only dust behind as he raced forward. We lived in its shadow, but rarely discussed his disease or the clock ticking on his way of life.

As the commercial building wrapped up, Rock called me one day from Big Sky. While he was a self-made man and had plenty of money, frugal is perhaps too kind a word to describe his way with spending. He was free with it for farm equipment, a new truck, some excellent hiking boots, maybe a new snowboard or with his kids, like an $800 inflatable vest so Nick wouldn't be buried in an avalanche, while I still paid my own way. My frivolous spending was contained to art and horses and tack. I could sell a horse or a saddle to get a different horse or new saddle, and I was fine with my small juggling act. The call from Big Sky was Rockey in stingy guy heaven. "Oh my God, Mag! They are cleaning up around the site and the dumpster is running over with dimensional lumber, huge timbers and siding and bundles of sheetrock! The whole building was a custom order, so the lumber yard won't take any returns. They're just throwing it away!" Three hours later, he pulled into the driveway with the lowboy trailer piled high with his found treasures and another trailer coming in right behind. He and some other guy unloaded the stuff into a bay of the shop, and he gave me an excited tour of all he'd found. He had called Jeff, the friend who owned the building, and asked if he could take the stuff away. Jeff, who was challenged just starting a lawnmower, said, "Hell yes! Saves me the dumpster fees."

Three months after that day, Rockey started a remodel of our pretty new home, adding a sunroom off the kitchen. His dumpster diving gave him all the supplies he needed to build this fabulous room, with his only cash layout being for shingles and two windows. He called on friends to place the huge microlam as a load-bearing beam between this room and the existing house and another half-monkey/half-man friend to shingle the very tall roof. I called it the dumpster room, and it was my favorite place in that house. The views were incredible, all overlooking the bare lands and beautiful hills to our south, east and west.

Rockey also had an odd habit or characteristic of forward motion with virtually no attention paid to looking back or considering consequences. I asked him once about his inability to think about consequences and he looked puzzled for minute.

"Consequences are always good, if you plan every detail thoroughly."

"What about the consequences to your health?" I asked.

His response was quick: "My health is good. I have a tremor and I get tired easily. My balance is a little shaky sometimes, but my health is good. I won't stop doing things to preserve something that isn't gone yet. I won't stop until I can't go forward anymore. Don't expect me to be careful, you know me better than that." And so I did, as he spelled out his next really big ideas.

They weren't meant to happen simultaneously, but the next big projects had some overlap. Rock had sold a strip mall that he owned with his partner, Tim, in Lino Lakes, Minnesota. They had never planned to do a commercial or retail site, but in a weird course of events, the commercial site was part of a small residential neighborhood he and Tim developed, and they were unable to ditch it. So they built a strip mall, and I handled the leases and contracts and managed the tenant issues for a few years. It provided a nice income, and when it sold, Rock invested the money with a stockbroker. When the economy started to bust in 2008 and people started talking about their losses in the stock market, he pulled all his money out before his investments turned to nothing. Now he had a pile of money and the wish to make it work for him, and of course he knew how to build things and how to make money off that.

We decided that we could put up two duplexes at the end of the driveway on our eighty-acre Gateway farm. With virtually no zoning restrictions, we designed the buildings, staked them out, got the septic and building permits and Rockey and his pals started digging the basements late that fall. Although we had been together for over fifteen years and married for seven, Rockey had not put my name on the deed for the Gateway farm. It took me a while to notice, but I did notice during this process when I went to the courthouse to apply for some permits for the buildings and they said, " You're not on this deed." The confrontation I started at home went as so many did in those years. He said he just forgot, and I said, "You forgot you had a wife?" He said, "No big deal, I'll fix it." I was silly enough to believe him. But the building of the duplexes continued through that winter. He flew off to Moscow in December for his third stem cell treatment, traveling once again with Jay, the stem cell doctor.

About the same time, we heard that the Bakken boom growing in North Dakota was creating serious housing shortages for all the roughnecks coming to work on wells. Sometime in early 2009, Rockey drove to Williston, North Dakota, to see if there were any building sites available to put up a couple of apartment buildings. Our idea was to build a couple buildings, eight units each with three-bedroom apartments, to fill the need for family housing in that town. The city planner was so overjoyed to hear Rockey's plan, they made him an amazing deal on a city lot and sent him back home with, "Whatever you need to get this done, we'll make it sail through." Once again, Rockey was in *wide-fucking-open* gear. He sent our building sketches off to a commercial draftsman in Minneapolis, drove there to pick up the plans and met that day with the commercial contracting company in Minneapolis who built the shopping center. Within a month, the plans were finalized, bids were rolling in and Rockey was making the first of hundreds of trips to Williston.

The construction of the duplexes on our home property was moving along well, and I moved into the job of calling subcontractors, ordering lighting, plumbing fixtures and flooring, and troubleshooting to be ready for occupancy by the end of the year. Of course, Rock was still the big boss, but I knew enough to be able to give him a progress report most nights, and the truth is, the subcontractors were good and kept up the pace without much nagging. Meanwhile, Rockey the human tornado was blazing through Williston and driving back and forth to Gateway, hauling every piece of excavating equipment he owned back to North Dakota as he insisted that he and Nick get the earthmoving part of the contract. He called his older son Rock Jr., and of course his old partner Tim was the other owner of the apartment project.

They got together to hammer out two holes in the frozen dirt of Williston. The diesel exhaust was thick in air on those ungodly cold days as they slammed back and forth trying to carve out what they needed to get the building started. I got lucky when I volunteered to set up the corporation in Montana for the ownership of the Williston apartment buildings, and I filed the paperwork and listed each of us individually as 25% owners. Rockey, me, Tim and his wife Pam. Fool me once, Rockey Goertz. No more assumptive ownership based on marriage for me. It was years before anyone noticed that I had gotten my name on a real estate deed.

The duplexes on our Gateway farm were ready for occupancy in January of 2010. I ran the advertising and got them rented quickly enough. There were very few country rentals outside of Bozeman and I kept the price just a smidge under the average rental price in order to fill them. I agreed to manage them as long as I was getting paid a management fee, since I wasn't an actual owner. Jab. What was there to argue with, 40% to a management company or 15% to me? Well played, Mag. Well played.

The frenetic pace Rockey was living was bound to take a toll on his health. His tremor was now present the whole length of his left arm. He could still quiet it by grabbing ahold of something, but that fix became less and less effective as the amount of involuntary movement increased. I asked him whether it was painful and he said, "Imagine lifting a small weight repeatedly all day, imagine the ache you might have after that." He was much more tired on those long days and not getting the rest he required. Rockey's left foot had a small drag and his balance became a tiny bit unsteady; both symptoms became more apparent at this ragged pace.

We traveled back to Minneapolis in early winter of 2010 with an appointment to see Dr. T, his neurologist at the University of Minnesota. Rockey told the doctor he was interested in DBS surgery, a very successful procedure being used on Parkinson's patients to control tremors. DBS stands for "deep brain stimulation" and is accomplished by implanting a neurotransmitter into a specific area of the brain—Rockey's would be placed on the right side of his brain for his left side tremor—with wires running from the transmitter under the skin, behind his ear, down his neck and chest and attached to a small battery placed under the skin of his torso. His symptoms were considered debilitating enough for him to be a candidate. In order to be approved for the surgery, he had to undergo a series of psychological tests to prove that he could accept a medical device implanted in his person. Once that was done, he was scheduled for the DBS surgery in May of 2010.

I made the flight reservations, making sure Rockey was in first class, left side window seat, because he still didn't want even strangers to see his tremor. The hotel I booked was within walking distance to the University of Minnesota hospital and a fabulous Thai restaurant. We settled into the room for a sleepless night before rising for the 5:00 a.m. admittance to the surgery center. As is the case with many types of brain surgery, the patient is conscious.

I was allowed to go back into the medical area for his surgical prep. The first thing they did was fit his head with a halo, an intercranial stabilization device, which was attached with screws into the scalp to insure stability. That was gross, but it didn't seem to cause him any pain. The neurosurgeon stopped in to review the procedure with him. She was a cold, brittle human being, and I remember thinking it was good she had a reputation for her excellent surgical skills, because her interpersonal skills were nonexistent. His halo would be attached to the surgical table to ensure stability and she would make a cut through his scalp to his skull. She would then use a circular drill bit to remove a small round piece of his skull into which they would implant the device and the wires would begin the long descent to the battery in his torso. I got hung up thinking about the drill and pressure of that in his head, so I missed some details, however when she told us that the small circle of bone removed would be referred to as the manhole, I snapped out of my nightmarish reverie, and I barked out a laugh. Rock laughed too, but the doctor most certainly did not. Picture him sitting there in a hospital bed with half his hair shaved, wearing this halo that was attached to his head with good-sized bolts, swabbed with orange antibacterial solution, while wearing the ridiculous hospital gown and nodding his understanding of the procedure.

She said once the wires were attached to the battery, she would begin to test the device. Rock would be asked to perform some verbal skills, a memory question or two, perhaps counting or the alphabet, all to prove that the placement hadn't disrupted any other brain activity. The last test would be to dial in the electrical stimulation to a level that would stop his tremor. Once all that was satisfactory, she would replace the manhole and close his scalp. He would enter the surgery with only a light sedation, in his case a small dose of Ativan, mostly to keep his heart rate and blood pressure within acceptable limits. I understood Rockey's need to try to control this uncontrollable disease, but this wouldn't be the last time I would marvel at his personal courage to undergo this awful procedure. I'm not sure I could have made that choice knowing what it entailed.

The results were astounding. His tremor was gone. Just gone. Rockey felt good, his overriding self-consciousness was gone, and his attitude had returned to being his indomitable self. For a while, we just lived our life. Parkinson's was not a player, not the most pressing thing to consider, not even a whisper of it except for his daily need for a nap. We maybe should have enjoyed it more because it was the last such respite there would be.

Fooking, North Dakota

After they finished the apartments in Williston in 2009, Rock couldn't resist throwing his hat in the ring to get a piece of the immense amount of earthwork being done in the area. The influx of workers for the oil and gas industry boom, and the export of all that extracted material, led to unprecedented growth in a large swath of western North Dakota. Single-family houses, apartment buildings, hospital expansions, hotels, and Walmart parking lots all required earth movers. There was a significant contingency of other subcontractors from Bozeman—plumbers, electricians, HVAC guys, and framers—who were all there trying to get a piece of this enormous pie. They kept in touch with each other, sending out alerts about bids on new projects. The area was exploding, but there was this short window of time when the number of subcontractors was still small, so they saw the potential to cash in. Rock bid almost everything he could get his mitts on, brought Nick and some of his pals from Montana and called on his son Rock Jr. from Minnesota to gather up a few guys for the crews. They took all the big equipment they owned—bulldozers, backhoes, bobcats and all the trailers to move them around. They rented big equipment locally as they needed it.

If housing was short for the roughnecks, it was almost impossible for the subcontractors. The RV parks and campgrounds were loaded to capacity and charging outrageous monthly fees, but the boys brought their fifth wheels, campers and RVs, happy to pay for the privilege of electric, water and septic hook-ups. Summers were hot, humid and mosquito-filled. North Dakota has a high water table and most of the earth they worked was an uncooperative kind of gumbo, making easy jobs take twice as long for all the times they had to redo. Winters were so bad they made the northerners question their heartiness. The bars were always packed, and the local law enforcement was overworked, understaffed and overwhelmed by the swarms of dirt and oil-covered men with too much cash looking to get drunk, get laid or fight. Rockey bought lots of beer in those months, hoping to keep the boys drinking safely in the campground rather than going off to town. Mostly it worked, but there were fights, drunken target shooting and sheriff's visits. Nobody got in real trouble while Rockey was there, but when he came back home, we were bound to get a late-night call from a sheriff or a jailer. As usual, when it came to his work or Nick-related things, I didn't say much, but I often wondered how the hell it could be worth all the trouble.

While he was in North Dakota, the work was extremely taxing on Rockey's body. Bad dirt, bad conditions, a frantic pace, in and out of big machines all day, the eight-hour one-way commute home and wild boys to keep corralled took a terrible toll on him. They only stayed about two years before excavators from all over the country poured in, diluting the amount of work available. The man that came home permanently from North Dakota was a diminished version of the one who first went there. He had stumbled over a rock and ruptured his Achilles tendon, torn his tricep off its anchor (both required surgery to repair), along with assorted other minor injuries. He was exhausted in a way that was difficult for him to ever recover from. After he came back, it didn't matter how much he slept, he was unable to repair whatever damage had been caused by those rough conditions and relentless pace. I harbored a grudge about North Dakota and Nick's need for taking

Rockey's last strong and healthy years. I also wondered what was so important to Rock that he gave it away so easily. He must have believed he had an unlimited supply of good years left.

Rockey continued to seek treatments for his Parkinson's as it insidiously kept up its theft of his person. He was still going to Russia once a year for stem cell treatments, and in 2011 returned to the University of Minnesota Hospital for a second Deep Brain Stimulation surgery, this time for the right-sided tremors that had appeared. Parkinson's is a two-sided disease, usually attacking one side of the brain at a time, until it's settled in firmly on both sides. The first DBS was a huge success, mitigating the tremors instantly and generally making him much more comfortable. The second one was as much a nightmare as the first one was a gift.

It was around Valentine's Day when he was admitted for surgical prep. This time, for some reason, the installation of the halo was hugely painful and caused Rock to feel apprehensive. Prior to wheeling him out for surgery, the surgeon came in and Rockey reminded her about the Ativan he'd been given the first time. She was brusque and unsympathetic as she told him he couldn't have it this time, causing him even more anxiety now that he knew what to expect from this procedure. We'll never know what went wrong that day—did her kid give her a hard time when she was leaving the house, perhaps an argument with her husband or a near traffic accident—but she wasn't on her game, and we both experienced an eerie feeling before they wheeled him into the surgical suite.

In the recovery room, Rock had much more pain than after the first DBS. Enough that his normally stoic self was agitated and demanding more relief. His speech was in terrible shape, his words had soft edges and little enunciation, and I had great difficulty understanding him. We had been scheduled to fly home the next day, but the surgeon asked him to stay for another day so they could tweak the settings and hopefully improve his speech. We made three trips to their office that day with no appreciable improvement in his ability to form words. They chalked the speech deficits up to post-surgical brain swelling, telling Rock it would get better and sent us home.

Several weeks later, it hadn't improved at all. I did some research and got him a prescription for speech therapy in Bozeman. He was fortunate to land with a kind, gifted therapist named Audra who rode horses and loved the backcountry. He worked hard and practiced her techniques diligently for a few months. He was beginning to see some improvement, and suddenly it all went away. The clarity of his speech became even worse than it had been right after the DBS. I wrote a letter to the surgeon, chronicling his progress and the setback. There were no accusations made, surely no threats of legal action, I just asked that she see him again to assess the placement of the neurotransmitter and perhaps look at a fix. Her office sent Rockey a letter, cc'd to the University Hospital attorneys, telling him he was no longer her patient, and he should seek another doctor. Rock was devastated because through this action, he was denied access to his fabulous neurologist, Dr. T. It was one thing for the hard-hearted neurosurgeon to cast him aside, but to lose the trusted Dr. T was a terrible loss.

About two years later, Rockey was encouraged by friends and family to pursue a lawsuit against the University Hospital and the surgeon. I told Rock I would organize this effort and be his voice, although I was not personally supportive of a lawsuit. My opinion was that it would take years of focus with a negative attitude and in the end, they would delay until Rockey was dead. I called an old friend of ours in Minneapolis and asked for recommendations for a good malpractice attorney. He sent a list of ten names. When I began to call these attorneys, I found that the top six were on retainer with the University of Minnesota Hospital. That left us to choose between lawyers who were considered below the B team. I made several attempts to secure letters from other doctors supporting the facts of Rockey's speech loss from the surgery. Ultimately, Rockey could see that we were small in a giant's fight and after months of trying to gather our own team, he said, "Let's just let it go."

Months passed and Audra did extensive research to try to figure out what caused the changes while we looked for a new neurological team. I researched neurology departments in Seattle, Salt Lake City and Denver. In order for a neurologist or neurosurgeon to treat or implant this type of neurotransmitter, they had to be certified by Medtronic, the device manufacturer. That narrowed the search because, at the time, the only one certified in any of those places, was in Seattle. However, after another conversation with Medtronic, they did tell me there was a team of neuro docs in Billings who were not only certified but had done a large volume of DBS surgeries. I was skeptical that a good team could be in Billings and recommended the Seattle team. Rockey liked the sound of the Billings doctors after I showed him my research, so I set up an appointment in Billings. The neurologist was Dr. Arturro Echeverri and the surgeon was Dr. Stuart Goodman. Echeverri was so delightful it was difficult not to feel immense relief at Rockey's good fortune in finding him.

Rockey told his sad tale, with me assisting when the doctor couldn't understand him. Echi, as we came to call him, thought Rock's sudden decline in speech was likely due to a post-surgical stroke. By this time, Rockey had completely turned off the new transmitter because he could feel electric impulses down his right side, and it was too distressing to leave it turned on. (The patient is sent home from DBS surgery with a small handheld gadget that can detect whether the transmitter is functioning, if the batteries are still good and turn it on or off.) Echi did some tests with his own computer and discovered that indeed the neurotransmitter was not functioning properly when it was turned on and recommended that his partner, Dr. Goodman, replace the device.

I was asked to get Rock's medical files from the University of

Minnesota, and they sent them directly to me by mistake. The file was huge, almost two inches thick, but I sent it on to Billings and we soon had an appointment to meet Dr. Goodman. He told us that replacement of neurotransmitters was a significant part of his practice, and he was the only doctor in the neighboring five states who was certified by Medtronic to install these transmitters. His practice partner, Dr Echeverri was certified to adjust the transmitter signals once it was in place. He had reviewed the file and believed that Rockey had good reason to have his hardware replaced, but it was unpredictable whether Rock would see any improvement to his speech. He offered an appointment in February, exactly one year to the day from the disastrous surgery. I requested a moment alone with Rock and asked him what he was thinking. He labored with his speech to tell me he was confident that we'd found the right guy and he wanted to go ahead. I waved the doctor back in and told him Rock was on board, and then we walked out feeling more hopeful than we had for months.

That was in November, and in December, Rockey made one more trip to Russia for stem cells. By this time, Jay had taken an apartment in Moscow because he traveled there often for other stem cell patients, so that became Rock's homebase for this trip. He had another allergic reaction to the transplant with a high fever and some delirium, but Jay treated him at the apartment, got the fever down, and Rockey was able to recover there without an extended hospital stay. (Rock went to Moscow five years in a row for stem cell transplants. There were never any remarkable changes and his disease continued on an expected trajectory.) This was nine years after his original diagnosis, and his condition was changing.

The neurotransmitters hid all outward signs of his tremors. I could feel the tremors deep in his body if I laid my hand on him as he slept, a continuous motion invisible to the human eye. His left foot drag had become significant enough that it required more energy to walk without stumbling and any distance over a third of a mile seemed too great. Because his torso had healed crooked after the mule disaster, he canted a bit to the left, further complicating his waning sense of balance. He was experiencing the muscle rigidity so common in Parkinson's patients, and it created a deep aching in his legs and arms. Massage helped relieve this pain, but the muscles would tighten up quickly when the session was over; nevertheless, he had weekly ninety-minute massages in hopes of retaining some suppleness.

The worst of all his symptoms was his speech, and he was horribly, painfully self-conscious about it. He had begun to withdraw socially, and our social life was meager to begin with. Rock was so incredibly unsure of himself that going to Stacey's, our famous local bar, for a burger or a steak sandwich became more challenging than he could bear. I tried to lighten his apprehension with things like, "We're old anyway. Nobody looks at old people in America." Or "Anybody we run into is a friend of yours, they won't judge you." None of my words helped, and eventually he became so anxious in a restaurant thinking people were staring at him for his weird gait, we quit trying. One evening before our food came, he looked at me with very wide eyes and said, "We have to go. Can we leave right now?" I threw some money down for the food we hadn't yet been served and helped him into my truck. After we'd gone a mile or so, he said, "I don't know what happened. My heart was racing, I couldn't catch my breath and I started seeing stars." I drove a little further and said, "Are you better now?" He nodded yes. I told him it sounded like a panic attack, and it would be okay. He was scared and said, "If that's what it was, I don't ever want one again. I'll just be staying home."

The few times we had dinner with friends in our home or someone else's, he was reluctant to speak, so it wasn't long before we stopped seeing anyone. He was comfortable with a couple of my friends, my faraway sister Kathy and a couple of his old pals, mostly neighbor Bob. I tried to discourage his desire for isolation, saying it might be too early to pull away, but this didn't help. He was very difficult to understand when he spoke, so I became his voice with anyone outside our tiny circle. When people asked him to repeat things, I could see in his eyes that it caused distress and embarrassment. He once said to me, "Well, it's kind of a waste of a good try. It's hard to form the words, I can only say things one way and saying them twice isn't going to make it easier to understand me." Although I had great empathy for him and his growing reluctance to talk because of the mechanical difficulty making words, it was the beginning of a long, lonely time for me.

He was still the restless man he'd always been, and now that he was losing his social abilities, he needed a new outlet for his fast-moving brain, so he began building furniture. The guy who had once fixed a broken coffee table for me with an eight-pound mall and a four-inch sheetrock screw left sticking out, set out to make fine furniture. He was self-taught, and by the time he put his saws away for good, he turned out some incredible pieces made with inlaid wood and elk horn drawer pulls. Even without speech, his fire of determination burned hot.

My role in our marriage was changing with each year he lived with Parkinson's and each silent theft the disease perpetrated. After the botched 2011 surgery, I became his voice for all but the most unguarded conversations with his friends. He was impossible to understand on the phone, so he mostly texted his kids and faraway friends. Neighbors looked at me with pleading eyes if they tried to talk with him, hoping I'd step in and relieve their discomfort. I never spoke for him unless he asked. I didn't finish his sentences and I never talked over him. He would ask with words or a gesture if he wanted me to speak for him, and I tried never to insinuate my voice into his conversations. This is when I began to notice how the medical community and many others treated Rockey. He walked with an ungainly sort of forward stumble that always made him look as if he were about to fall. Not only were his words muddy, but his voice had grown so soft, even if he had enunciated, he was nearly impossible to hear unless a person stood very close or, like me, tried to read his lips.

There had also been another development in his ability to communicate. In a normal conversation with someone, there is a timing to speaking and responding. If you and I were talking, I would say something, and in a second or two you would respond. Conversations with Rockey now had a significant delay, sometimes more than ten seconds before he could utter a response. I worked on self-control to try to let him speak in his own time. I kept reminding myself how I hated to be talked over or interrupted and thought how magnified that bad feeling would be for someone struggling to talk. I didn't want to make it harder for him, but I found it to be a difficult adjustment and fought hard against the impulse to rush him.

His driver's license needed to be renewed, and he made an appointment to go to the Montana license renewal office in Bozeman. He didn't think he needed my help, because he didn't expect to have to talk much, just get a new photo and take the eye exam. His examiner took the photo, did the eye exam and led him to her desk for a signature and payment. She then said loudly, "Something is wrong with you. You talk funny and you can't walk right. Stand up." He stood and said quietly that he had Parkinson's but there was no reason he couldn't drive. She kept on remarking about his speech, grabbed his hands and pulled him forward. He stumbled but did not fall and sat back down. She continued to remark on his poor speech and said she didn't feel she could renew his license. He asked why and she said, "Well, you can't talk." He asked her to show him where good speech was required to drive in Montana, and she told him to leave and that she had determined he was medically unfit to renew his license.

When he got home and told me, I was beyond furious. I first called the Director of the Motor Vehicle Department in Helena and asked what this examiner's medical qualifications might be along with some of my best swear words. He made the mistake of telling me to calm down. I then began calling Rockey's doctors, all of them, asking them to immediately flood this MVD office with letters explaining why his speech condition had absolutely no bearing on the motor skills required to be a safe driver. I called the Director back and demanded, with a few more swear words, that he provide me proof of the examiner's medical qualifications to make this medical decision about my husband. I told him he might want to check his fax machine as I had gotten four calls back from doctors saying they had already faxed the office of licenses in Helena.

I then called his speech therapist, who may have been angrier than I was. She not only wrote a letter, she actually drove down and delivered it personally with a scathing rebuke to the examiner who had humiliated Rockey. Next on my list was Senator Jon Tester's office where I used fewer swear words and pleaded for immediate help, using words like discrimination against a disabled person. Poor Rockey always hated hearing me speak tough to people to get him the services he needed, usually medical facilities, but this day his sad face smiled as I dialed office after office tearing around the state on his behalf, until the phone started to ring back. By late afternoon, the Director who told me to calm down called to apologize, and granted Rockey a five-year renewal of his license. I asked Rock if he wanted to talk to him and he shook his head. I told the man this was great, but I also expected a formal letter of apology to Rockey from the overzealous examiner by the end of the week. Rock got that letter and one from the Director in Helena as well as a wonderful letter from Jon Tester's office making sure Rockey had gotten a satisfactory resolution to the problem. Yay for the doctors and Senator Tester. Yay for me. I was exhausted after expending all that indignance.

Meanwhile, Rockey continued to archery elk hunt. In August, he would set up a target by the driveway and spray paint marks on the ground at thirty, forty, fifty and sixty yards. Every year I held my breath a little, hoping this wasn't the year he wouldn't be able to shoot his bow. Every year he'd come back in the house beaming that he was still a deadeye shot. The big wall tent camps were now much closer and usually set up within easy access to the main trail.

They also didn't happen to be anywhere near where elk lived, so after helping him set up that big tent a couple years in a row, he decided to let that practice go. As usual, he didn't say much about what was in his heart after that decision, but I imagined that of all the losses he suffered, letting go of horse packing caused the greatest heartbreak.

Check-in for his replacement DBS surgery was at 5:30 a.m. I noticed right away a difference in the staff at St. Vincent's when compared to the U of M Hospital. The pace was less frenetic, they made more eye contact during the intake procedures, generally took a bit of time for some kindness toward Rockey, and each person we talked to made sure they wrote down my name and phone number. A Medtronic representative was always present for the implant of any of its devices, and it was she who took us from the waiting room back to the surgical prep area. By this third DBS, the prep routine was familiar, and I took a walk around the halls while they attached the halo to his head. I understood that this surgery was necessary, but once again was blown away by the courage it took for him to agree to this, to allow them to drill a hole in his head while he was awake.

Dr Goodman stopped in before they took Rockey away. He went over the procedure again and added that this one may take longer than the two previous DBS surgeries. He would take out the older transmitter, determine the placement of the new one and check the wires, which he planned to replace in another surgery a few weeks down the road. He touched my arm and said, "We'll be okay and we will both see you in a while. Get out of here and go for a walk or something. I think you might spend too much time in places like this." He brightened then and asked if I brought the dogs. I said, "Of course. They're in my truck." He then told me how to find a cool place to have a little adventure with them. I squeezed his arm and said "Thanks, I'll do just that. Do your best, Doc!" smiling at the kind thought from a fellow dog lover. I gave Rock a kiss, walked down a hallway and down one more then quickly down a flight of stairs, sprinting out the front door and happily breathing in the cold fresh air of outside.

Fortified with a few miles in the fresh air, talking and hiking with my good dogs and a tall triple latte, I walked slowly into the hospital a few hours later. Back up the stairs and down two long hallways, I found the cluster of hospital chairs and gave my name to the lady at the desk and sat down to wait.

More time than felt right had passed and some worry settled into my mind when I looked up and saw Dr. Goodman striding toward me. He sat next to me and said, "He's all right, but it was more complicated than I anticipated, so we were in there a little longer than I like. The old transmitter had been implanted in a dangerous part of the brain and the previous surgeon had used a very aggressive approach, plus she used a newer smaller model of transmitter that doesn't have as sure a track record as the one I use. When I removed it, I found the damage to his speech center and I'm sorry, but there was nothing I could do to fix that, it was necrotic. I decided it would be less trauma for Rockey to stay a little longer today than to return in a few weeks, so I also ran the new wires to the battery. I feel like we will have a much more successful implant than the one he came in with, but you have to understand, this was difficult surgery because of the extra work we did and the time it took. He's strong enough to come out of it okay, but his recovery will likely not be as easy as with the others. Because of the wire work, he was under anesthesia quite a while. What questions can I answer for you?"

I stared off for a moment then looked at him and asked, "Does Rockey know you couldn't fix his speech?"

The doc said, "No. Well, he won't remember that part anyway. But I did not say it definitively while he was on the table. We're going to keep him in recovery for another hour or two until he starts to come around, then we'll take him to ICU for the night. He's pretty out of it, so if you want you can just wait for us to move him." I asked if Rock was combative right now and the doctor said, "Some, when he starts to wake up, but he's still drifting back to sleep." He asked me if Rock was usually good with anesthesia.

"He used to be, but recently it's been taking him much longer to come out of it and he's pretty loony for a while. I'll skip this part if you think he's okay."

Goodman laughed and said that was fine. He gently shook my hand and said, "He's a lucky man to have you in his corner. Take all the time you need. We've got him now. Get lost. I will stay around, and I'll call you when we move him to ICU. We'll probably release him tomorrow and he'll be back in your hands again."

My eyes teared up as I stood and zipped my coat, heading down the long hallways and stairs again to take a big gulp of the fresh crisp air outside. I didn't go far. Just took the dogs and walked the streets of the neighborhoods near the hospital trying to sort out all the doctor had told me. Soon enough, he called and said Rock was in his room.

I had to pick up a pass to be admitted into the ICU and some-one guided me to Rockey. He looked pretty good but was experi-encing a lot of pain. His nurse Kathy was a gem. She asked what had been successful for Rock in the past to treat pain. I told her what I thought would work best, feeling amazed that a nurse was open enough to ask what had been successful before, and within a couple hours, he was finally losing that pinched look around his eyes. Kathy told him when he was stable, he could sit in the easy chair in his room to get some relief from the hard hospital bed. I helped him get there, arranging his IV stand and tubes and got out the menu for him to choose some dinner. He looked at me with a sad face after all the arranging was complete and said, "Oh geez, sorry, now I have to pee." I laughed as I moved all his tubes again and helped him stand and handed him the bottle and disappeared behind the curtain. Moments passed and I heard an odd sound and said, "Are you okay?" I thought I heard a garbled reply and it sounded like the bed was moving. I whipped back the curtain to find him falling with his upper body still on the bed. His arms were clutched to his chest, his face in a terrible grimace and he seemed to be trying to curl up as he slid off the bed toward the floor. I bent down and grabbed his shoulders, cupping his bandaged head with one hand and pulled him into my chest so he wouldn't hit his already wounded head. His whole body was rigid, it seemed like every muscle flexed and I had a hard time holding his head to me to protect it. I called out, "Kathy, Help!"

The next few minutes are full of blurry action, but suddenly there were many hands, some lifting and supporting Rockey, some helping me to stand while I continued to cradle his head to my chest. Someone peeled my arms off Rock as they swiftly but gently laid him on his bed. There may have been four people helping him, checking vitals, and someone kept shouting "Rockne! Rockne! Can you hear me?" I quietly said, "His name is Rockey. Only his mom calls him Rockne," as I pressed my back against the wall trying to stay out of the way. He didn't know his name; he couldn't squeeze their finger. Rock couldn't focus his eyes and he had no response to pain stimulus. Just as suddenly as they all appeared, they unlocked the bed wheels and hurriedly pushed him out of the room. "Where are you taking him?" I said. "To get a scan to see if there is a bleed," someone said over their shoulder as they raced away.

Thinking I was alone, I slid to the floor and pulled my knees up tight to my chest, wrapped my arms around my legs and laid my head on my knees and tried to catch my breath. My heart was pounding, my breathing was ragged and I felt a little dizzy. I sat like that for what seemed like a nanosecond when a gentle hand touched my shoulder and a soft voice said, "Maggie, are you okay?" The funniest thought flew into my brain, and I said, "Wow! That's the first time somebody remembered my name." I looked up and it was Kathy, and her smile was warm as she said, "First, who could ever forget you? You're a pretty important player in this thing." I laughed and told her I was okay … just a little adrenaline overload for the old broad.

She sat me in the nice chair, pulled out the footrest and handed me a bottle of water. She said, "Just sit there and take a minute. They will all be back too soon."

It was only a few minutes before they wheeled him back in, and a young man stood at his head and started shouting again. I stood and reached across Rockey and touched the man on his arm. He looked at me and I said, "Let me try." I bent in very close, took Rockey's hand and pressed my chest against his arm, holding his hand by my face and whispered, "Rock, I'm here and all these nurses and doctors are here to help you. I'm right here and you are safe." I stroked his face and said the same thing again. The young man, who I could now read on his badge was a doctor, started to interrupt to hurry us along. I gave him the stink eye and said through clenched teeth, "Maybe back up, stop shouting and give us a minute."

I continued to say Rockey's name, my name and that he was doing okay and was safe as he stared with wide eyes at some noth-ingness far away. Eventually I asked him if he could look at me. He turned his head with incredible slowness, but he turned it the wrong way. I asked again and very gently took his chin in my hand and turned his head to me. He looked so afraid my heart nearly broke, and I kept talking softly—his name, my name, safe. I finally told him he had fainted, and he was okay, but the doctor wanted to check a few things and I'd be close by. I nodded to the doctor and said, "No more yelling, please, he can hear you," and I stepped out to speak to Kathy. She quickly told me the scan found no brain bleed and that what he had experienced was a series of intense seizures. Just then my phone buzzed, and it was Dr. Goodman. He told me he'd seen the scan and repeated what Kathy had just said, adding that seizures are a risk when they are messing in the brain for a long period of time. I asked if Rock could come back from this and he said, "I think so, but it will take some time because the surgery and his Parkinson's complicates that healing." He said he'd see me tomorrow and we hung up.

. . .

Back in the room, Rockey had finally responded to pain stimulus, but couldn't do anything else yet, and he certainly could not speak. I sort of budged my way through the clot of people around his bed and resumed my position, taking his hand in mine. His eyes still carried that fear and I kept trying to reassure him. His vitals were stable, and the crowd thinned out until it was just Rock and me. Eventually, he squeezed my hand and I asked him to wiggle one foot, then the other. I felt like he could understand me, and I guessed he was freaking out about not being able to speak. Hoping that he wouldn't remember this whole episode, I repeated the lie about fainting, thinking the word seizure would scare him even more. I talked a little BS about post-surgical stuff, making it up as I went along, and told him that he just had to get the anesthesia out his system and he'd be able to talk again by morning. He seemed to be getting sleepy and I decided to make my move. I gave him a kiss, told him to try to sleep and that I'd be back in the morning. I stopped by the nurses' station and let them in on what I'd told Rockey, made sure they had my number and slipped away for what was left of the night.

The area by the hospital was a better neighborhood for a dog walk than near the hotel, and I told the dogs they better hurry up as I got them out of the truck one more time. Back at the hotel, I got a bag of yucky Sun Chips out of the vending machine for my day's nourishment, let the dogs in the room and stripped off the clothes that I felt as if I'd been wearing forever and stood weeping in the shower as I let the water wash away the stink of fear and the hospital. The sights, sounds and information of the day swirled around in my head. I felt too exhausted to light on anything for long. One thought, one feeling was persistent. I had seen Rockey through some awful things that caused him great physical pain and giant waves of worry. Right now, in this hotel room still wet from the shower, I thought with certainty that the very worst thing I had ever seen was the fear in his eyes after that seizure. I knew how to help him manage pain and I'd grown skilled at diminishing his worries, but I didn't think I possessed the tools to be able to take away that fear, and it felt like a rip in my heart.

I awoke feeling like shit, got dressed, packed up our stuff, loaded the dogs, grabbed a giant coffee and found a quiet place to let the dogs run a little. I feared that, even considering yesterday's events, they would release Rockey to go home. I didn't have much hurry left in me as I made my way down the hallways and past the flock of hospital chairs. I waved my badge and entered the ICU and kind of snuck up to peer around the entrance to his room. He was sitting up, dozing, so I went back to the nurses' station for any update. New day, new people, and they told me Rock had been heavily sedated, so the night had been quiet, and that Dr. Goodman should be around anytime. I tiptoed back into his room and sat quietly in the recliner waiting for a new day of chaos to begin.

When Goodman arrived, he caught my attention and motioned me out into the hallway before waking Rockey. He said he'd be releasing Rock and he was prescribing antiseizure medications and that these meds would act like sedation for Rockey at first. Dr. Goodman stressed the importance of correct dosage and delivering that dosage on time as we gradually stepped that dosage up over the next two weeks. He believed the total loss of speech was from the seizure and that he should recover at least the muddled speech he had when he arrived. I was to keep him as quiet and still as possible for three days and then let him walk around the house a little. Rockey was never to be unattended and absolutely never to try to walk unattended. He couldn't say how long this supervision would be necessary but that after a week, if I thought his balance was good enough, I could take him for short walks outside. He was scheduled to come back and see Dr. Goodman in three weeks.

. . .

Back in the room, Dr. Goodman explained to Rockey what was happening in a simpler version of what he told me. As a person who has worn every emotion on my face for my whole life, I found myself working hard at keeping a poker face. I knew wordless Rockey would take any cues he could find from my expressions, and my goal was to give him nothing but calm. After the crazy night before, this was all oddly quiet. The doctor asked Rock if he had any questions and they both looked to me. I took Rock's hand, and he shook his head and one tear rolled down his face. A couple of hours later, they wheeled him down to the emergency exit, helped him into my truck and we headed home to Gateway.

Post Seizure

This wouldn't be the last time I drove too fast on winter roads
trying to get a broken Rockey back home. Something in this hospital stay had heightened his sensitivity to light and sound. With
the radio playing softly, he kept trying to figure out the volume. I
was driving 85 mph and trying hard not to pay attention to whatever he was doing, but finally he slapped the dashboard, and I said,
"What, Rock? Do you want it louder or off?" His hand made a
horizontal sliding motion and I hit the button to turn it off. I got a
thumbs up from him. It dawned on me that we had already had a
few of these hand motion conversations in the past year, although
this situation was more acute. Next, even with his ever-present
sunglasses on, the low-slung, bright sun reflecting off the snow
was bothering his eyes. He couldn't tell me with words, but he kept
messing with the inadequate visor on the passenger side and he
seemed to be wearing a grimace of pain. I pulled off the freeway
down an exit ramp and drove halfway up on the entrance ramp
and put it in park. I hopped into the back and dug around under
the seat pulling out a backpack of weird things I always carried.

Bingo, I found a well-used but clean dish towel, shook a little dog hair out of it, got back in the driver's seat and hung the towel over his visor for better sun protection. He didn't speak but reclined the seat, put his bandaged head back and fell asleep. I was grateful for a tiny win in this new wordless world.

The hospital was 168 miles from our house, two hours and forty-five minutes if everything went well. Big Timber was close to the halfway mark and also the eastern edge of the *Super Big Wind Tunnel* as I liked to call it, where it's not uncommon to find winds in the 40 mph range for the next fifty miles. I had just started to feel the crosswinds pushing my truck a little and Rock hit my arm with the back of his hand. I looked over with my eyebrows raised and he pointed to his crotch. I let out a chuckle and said, "Oh no, you've got to pee? We're in the Wind Tunnel." And my chuckle turned into a laugh as he gave a lopsided grin and made a big shrug with his hands. Having driven this highway many times on the big trip from Minnesota, I knew the best exit to take for a roadside pee for Rockey, who'd had prostate trouble for at least a dozen years. I exited down a Ranch Road access exit and turned onto a little dirt road and once again put it in park. I unbuckled his seat belt, and the wind caught the door as he opened it. Rock was already unzipping as I shouted, "Step ahead or it will blow back into the truck!" He took a bumbling step forward, hanging on to the door with his left hand while, with my eyes closed, and laughing softly, I gently banged my head on the headrest saying, "Oh god, oh god, oh god." One of the dogs nudged its head against mine as if to give comfort. We were only halfway home.

It was uneventful the rest of the way. I had a small supply of the prescriptions he would need but didn't want to stop at the pharmacy on our way through Bozeman and make him wait. We got in the house, and I helped him get his shoes off and head toward relaxing. I asked him, "Chair or bed?" and he pointed to his chair. He sat and patted the arm of the chair and looked puzzled, and I took a wild guess and moved his hand to the electric recline button. The chair whirred as it laid back a little and his feet came up. I covered him with a throw, got him some ice water and sat down near him. I picked up the TV remote and turned it on and handed Rock the remote. He looked at it, shook his head, and handed it back with another shrug. This wasn't that alarming, as his TV management skills had been less adept. I found something for him to watch and he had one more request. He made a V with his fingers and motioned to his face. I went to his nightstand and got him one Kool cigarette. This weird guy had been smoking one Kool cigarette a day since long before I met him. At night. He called it his goodnight cigarette and told me that when he was young and wanted to quit smoking, he decided he could have one cigarette a day, but he had to choose the most important one in order to make it work. It was the goodnight smoke. He had scary self-discipline on some things.

He finished the cigarette, laid that chair all the way back and fell into a long, deep sleep. I put on a coat and sat on the cold concrete front steps and tried to figure out what this was going to be like.

The antiseizure drugs seemed powerful from my perspective. By the third day home, Rock was regaining some speech although it was mushy, and he gave up quickly if I misunderstood. I asked him if it was physically difficult to form the words or if he couldn't think of the word he wanted. He shook his head and said, "No," and he picked up the bottle of drugs and said, "I'm dopey." I had been doling out more information to him about what happened, so he understood he'd had a seizure, but I hadn't explained much about the meds. I told him he was going to have to be on them for at least a few weeks and that quitting too soon increased his risk of another seizure. Of course, he said, "Let's quit them." I was patient as I explained again, this time using more of the dire warnings the doctor had given me. That the meds effectively quieted the electrical storm his brain wanted to produce, that another storm could impact him badly and permanently, that the surgery was a success, but it was very, very hard on him as allowing someone to dig around in your brain with a spoon can be. That was one of my favorite brain surgery lines and it made him laugh every time. I was adamant that he stay on the antiseizure meds and the consequences of quitting were not something we could live with.

It was a slow recovery. Rockey hated the heaviness and slowness he felt from the meds. He couldn't drive, he slept a lot, he had several smaller seizures and likely some small strokes, and each time they increased the medication, and each time I didn't tell him. But by May he was able to begin to wean off these drugs, and by July he was doing as well as he would ever do. The new neurotransmitter was doing its job in controlling his tremors and the speech deficit that he had going into that surgery remained the same.

July was haying time. We have about fifty acres of premium alfalfa/grass mixed hay that we mostly sell and ten acres of pure grass hay that I keep and feed to my horses and sheep. Rock had been fortunate to have the weather on his side more years than not, and he had a reputation for good hay with no weeds. The act of haying was beginning to be too damn much for him. Too many days, too many times in and out of the tractor or the swather. The frustration of the inevitable breakdown almost caused him to fall apart, and these were all things that everyone who made hay experienced. He and I had done all of it ourselves for a long time and it was a hard sell to convince him that we needed help. The help wouldn't come that year, but he and good neighbor Bob found a way to work together that lightened the load for a few years in the future.

I reluctantly helped Rockey set up an elk camp that fall. It was only a couple mile ride from the trailhead, and he got lost when we rode in to set up the tent. I hadn't been there yet, and he kept asking me where we might have missed the turn. His confusion worried me when I considered him being out here at night and alone, but it

73

wasn't very high or rough country and was well-used and I figured if he stayed lost, eventually he would run into a trail that could take him out. We rode way too far, and I finally convinced him we needed to turn around and find the side trail we had missed. The trip took us four hours longer than it should have, and by the time we found the right spot, the day was long and poor Rockey was spent. I was tired, too, but I didn't want to come back to help on another day, so I started trying to put up the wall tent alone as I had suggested he lay down for a bit. I almost had it up and secure until the ridge pole got crooked and collapsed on my head. I didn't scream, but there was plenty of swearing as I tried to crawl out of the heavy mess I had made. The pole had cut my head and I didn't want Rock to feel responsible, so I wrapped a bandana on the cut and smashed my hat down on top of it to stem the bleeding. It was only about a two-inch cut and not very deep, but head cuts bleed a lot. The part of this that stands out in my mind is that I was reluctant to go in the first place and that I didn't want to return on a second day to finish the setup. Our back country time had always been the place where everything was all right and I truly loved these trips. Yes, it was a physically demanding pastime, but worth every sore muscle in my mind. I'm short but tough and was very strong in those days, but I couldn't set up this camp by myself without great difficulty. As a prime example, I just couldn't lift that ridge pole high enough, even with my arms fully extended. Rockey's diminishing strength and stamina, the loss of his balance and core strength and the fact that he just didn't see things clearly—like the order of the poles to put up that giant tent—insured the backcountry experience had devolved into shitty time. He yelled at me when he couldn't command his body to do what we needed. He yelled at me for going too fast. He yelled at me for everything, and I hated every minute of this thing that I had once loved so much. Setting up while he napped seemed to be a good way to avoid all the yelling.

So, with my bloody head disguised, I took another whack at the ridgepole. I balanced one end on a fat, punky log that I could use as a lever to get it to its proper height. The punky log was sturdy enough, but the rot made it light enough for me to lift. Back and forth from one end to the other, inching it higher and higher, set the corners and, voila, I got it done. But I wasn't coming back to this camp.

When Rockey finally stirred, he was surprised I had gotten the tent up. He dragged the kitchen packs and a few more things inside and off we went back down to the trailhead. About six weeks later, he went in alone to strike the camp and had the packs loaded up on Pete and was riding Poncho, both steady, calm creatures. Quite suddenly, on a bit of a cliff ledge, Poncho started to rear and dance. When Poncho stumbled back a couple of steps, he bumped Pete hard enough that Pete went over the edge and tumbled down about thirty feet while the packs went flying. Rock told me he dismounted and stood there staring down at Pete for a minute, wondering what to do next. Good old Pete stood up, shook himself and started to walk up a less steep incline back to the trail. Rockey rode Poncho forward and when he got to the flatter spot that Pete was heading for, he tied them both to a tree and tried to descend to the packs. Steep and stumbly ground made him cautious, but when he got to the packs, he found all the clips needed to attach it to the packsaddle were broken. Each pack was about 125 pounds, and he couldn't stand to leave them, so he started to drag them, one at a time, closer to the trail. He got one closer and set it under a tree and was in the process of moving the second when he heard voices. He looked and saw four young men walking down the trail.

They looked down at Rock and said, "Hey man, can you use some help?"

"Well yeah, I sure could," he answered in his slow way.

They asked what he was trying to do, and one of the young guys said, "That parking lot isn't very far, how about if we just carry them out for you?"

In Rock's new state of emotional rawness, he told me it was all he could do to not cry, and he said, "I'd be grateful for any help right now." He said he didn't know if they could understand his words, but he nodded to them as well.

Rock rode ahead of them and they each grabbed one end of the big packs walking effortlessly down the trail. At the trailer, Rockey got off Poncho and tied both horse and mule to the trailer and showed the young guys where to put the packs. They were MSU students out looking for a good trout lake and Rock was happy to direct them. He dug in his wallet and found an old, folded $100 bill and handed it to one of the guys, saying, "I've been saving this for an emergency, and I think this qualifies. Can't thank you enough." He watched the strong young men stride away with smiles and swinging arms and stumbled into his truck, laid his head on the steering wheel and wept for what he would never be again. He didn't tell me the story for a few weeks. I think he was waiting to tell me until he could relate it without all the emotion he felt. I still thought it was a powerful encounter for him and a lucky one, too.

The big wall tent camps were now much closer and usually set up within easy access to the main trail. They also didn't happen to be anywhere near where elk lived, so after helping him set up that big tent a couple years in a row and after the pack wreck incident, he decided to let that practice go. As usual, he didn't say much about what was in his heart after that decision, but I imagined that it was a huge loss.

The year 2013 was an angry and lonely year. Rockey was angry for all his body's betrayals, and I was lonely because he was so fully immersed in being that guy. His speech was and always would be difficult—difficult to understand and difficult for him to produce. He felt sorry for himself most all the time, not that anyone could blame him, but it's an ugly quality all day, every day. He couldn't make his hands do what he wanted anymore, like fit a wrench onto a bolt or reach into a piece of equipment and grab hold of that wire he could see. I could hear him throwing things and roaring if I happened to walk anywhere near his shop. He didn't drive any big equipment anymore, because he was just too dangerous to have on a job site. His reflexes were slow and unpredictable. It was too easy for him to cause a machine to lurch forward or not be able to stop one quickly enough. I told Nick I didn't think it was safe to let Rock drive the big trailers carrying equipment up the canyon anymore. The road to Big Sky kills enough people every year without encouraging a compromised guy to drive 70,000 pounds around all those curves. Nick agreed and said it was scary to watch Rockey moving dirt so we agreed Nick would assign him all the stick work. Of course, neither Nick nor I wanted to be the one to tell Rockey he was dangerous, so we decided this indirect plan would work for now. Stick work meant he would take measurements, figure out the grading plan and how much dirt would be removed or added and put marking sticks in all the right places on a job site. He couldn't kill anybody with lath and hot pink survey tape, and he got to boss around the operators, so it wasn't all bad for him.

Rockey's ability to function independently was adequate in 2013. I was happy to spend my days out of his circle of influence, riding my horse and hiking big miles discovering new places of wonder. Sometime in late winter, he decided he wanted to get his knee fixed. He'd had several arthroscopic procedures years before and somehow determined that he needed another. We first went to what I'll call the East Side Orthopedic Clinic. I went along to most of his doctor appointments now because he was unable to recall or report what happened in these appointments. He was X-rayed and examined, and the doctor determined that there wasn't much wrong with that knee and suggested Rock just wear a flexible brace. Rockey argued the best he could, and I remained silent. The doctor good-naturedly said, "Sorry, Mr. Goertz. I think there wouldn't be much benefit for you. The knee isn't in bad enough shape to warrant a surgical procedure right now."

Rock was silent as he stalked off to my truck and he grumbled all the way home. A few weeks later, he wanted me to get him an appointment with a surgeon in what I will call West Side Orthopedics. Again, he was X-rayed and examined, but this doctor said, "Sure," and scheduled the procedure, an arthroscopic meniscus repair, for two weeks out. This was a day surgery and so the recovery wasn't awful, except for the fact that his walking was impaired to begin with. He went to physical therapy and was pronounced healed after some time. He was unhappy with the results, and I must admit, I wasn't paying keen attention to his rehab. Rockey wanted to go in and talk to the surgeon and decided to go without me. He came home angry with the doctor because the doctor said there was nothing wrong. I still was only half-listening and probably nodded at the appropriate times and made sympathetic sounds. His perpetually angry state had made it easy for me to disengage because it seemed he just wanted to rage about everything. A few weeks later, he scheduled a repeat visit with this same surgeon and wanted me to come along to witness how he was being dismissed.

This time the surgeon was defensive and said, "What do you want? There is nothing wrong with your knee," and he showed us all the images.

Rockey yelled at the doctor, "You were supposed to make me walk again!"

The doctor yelled back, "I fixed your knee!"

Every alarm bell in my head went off. The doctor was red-faced. Rockey was red-faced. And I just sat there with my practiced poker face. I looked into the doctor's eyes and waited a beat. I stood up and touched Rock's sleeve and said, "Come on, Rock. It's time to go."

He raged all the way home, and I didn't hear much of it. What I heard him say to the doctor was alarming to me, but I knew I needed to think it through and process it sometime when he wasn't yelling right next to me. The weeks slipped by into summer and soon enough, he brought up the knee surgery again. He wanted a redo.

I said, "The first clinic turned you away because it wasn't bad enough to require surgery. You got the second to do the surgery you wanted and now it's fixed. I'm not sure what it is you're look-ing for."

He looked pissed. He said, "If it was fixed, I'd be able to walk."

I paused for minute and said, "Rock, you can't walk because you have Parkinson's. Sweetie, nobody can fix that."

He bellowed, "NOOOOO!" He took two steps toward me and pushed me hard. I flew backwards and slammed into a wall and my feet slid out from under me.

I scrabbled for purchase, got to my feet and ran for the door thanking god he was so slow. I hollered for the dogs, and we all took off running down the driveway. I could hear him starting up the ATV so I started crossing fences knowing he would have to stop to open gates and thinking if I got to the canal and crossed it, he couldn't get to me. Of course, the dogs just thought we were going swimming, so they were happily running along. We crossed the canal easily because it was only three feet deep in mid-sum mer and I started heading south on the trail the ditch rider used. There was a road Rock could drive to catch me if he drove out to the highway and came toward me, but I knew this piece of land much better than Rockey did and hurried along to a big gully with tons of trees for cover. Relieved to be out of sight, we traveled the gully for a while and then I climbed up to get a view. I saw Rockey had traded the ATV for his pickup and was coming up the lane. I wasn't scared anymore because I knew he couldn't see me, he didn't even know this gully was here, and I had been hiking this neigh-bor's ranch for years. I sat on my perch and watched him leave, and I could see him turn up our driveway.

I didn't have a plan, and I wasn't afraid for my person anymore, but I didn't feel like going back yet, so we just stayed low and kept hiking higher on the ranch. The gully ran parallel to our farm but about three quarters of a mile away. I knew well when I would reach the place in the gully where no one could see me when I popped out. I had run out of the house wearing some water sandals. Although they stayed tightly strapped to my feet, they were hardly working in my favor by now and my bare ankles were scratched to bits. It would be gentler country as I crossed the big wide open over soft prairie grass. It happened to be the best choice my scrambled brain could make. As soon as I entered the tall grass, my heart slowed, my face relaxed and I could breathe deeply again. We walked slowly through this grass and after a little way, I called the dogs to me and sat down. I laid back in the tall grass and could see a beautiful piece of blue Montana sky and my pals laid down beside me. I thought about this spot, how the big wide open had soothed me so quickly and how lucky I was to feel that. I had hurried up the nasty gully with my tears, my rage, my scraped-up ankles and heart-pounding fear. I could feel that dark stuff leaving me, except for the scraped-up ankles. As I stared up, I thought through "being stuck" and talked to myself and the dogs about not being stuck. "I won't live with a violent person." Dogs' tails wagged. "And I won't be stuck." More wagging. "I have no idea what that means, but I'm going with the idea for now."

After a bit more self-talk, the dogs and I kept walking across this top line of the ranch until our farm came clearly into view. We sat again and I watched the place, seeing whether there was any activity. I thought it was kind of creepy to know that if I had some binoculars, I might be able to see into my house from way up here. I didn't have a watch or my phone, but I knew we'd been gone for a couple hours. While I was sitting there, I wondered, when you're amped up because of anger or because of fear, does one of those emotions settle down faster than the other?

My fear was mostly gone, and I wondered whether Rockey's anger was too. I stood and started walking toward the house a little less than a mile away. I did feel some apprehension the closer I got, but I walked up the front steps and peered through the screen door. He was sitting in his chair staring at a silent TV. I said, "Hey, is it safe to come in?" He looked at me with the saddest face and started to get out of the chair. I opened the door, held up my hand and said, "No, stay put. I'll come over there." I walked around the stairwell, so I didn't have to come too close to him and sat at the far end of the couch. He was sorry. He was so, so sorry. I believe he was. I also knew that a threshold had been crossed, that he had somehow moved into a state of denial which allowed him to think that somewhere, someone could do a surgery that would restore his ability to move fluidly. If he didn't believe it was the Parkinson's, then somebody could fix it. In that moment, I couldn't have known how that might impact him or us. I just thought that the holes in his brain were causing big trouble with his ability to reason. Pushing me that hard was not who he was, not who he had been. I might be able to forgive it, but I knew I certainly could not forget it, and it colored how I saw him for the rest of our days together.

The next day, I made a getaway bag. In this bag, I put my birth certificate, my insurance papers, my passport, Rockey's will, the title to my truck and trailer, the registration papers for my horses and $1,000 cash. I also put some extra jeans, shirts, a couple coats and hats—because it's Montana and you never know. I shoved extra boots, rain gear and socks under the seat of the truck. My sleeping bag and pillow got smashed into the smallest bag I could fit them into and both bags stayed in my truck. I started parking my truck outside and backed into my space. I wasn't stuck. Well, at least I wasn't stuck without a change of clothes.

The Wounds

Things felt bruised, not physically but in my heart, maybe my spirit, for a long time. I discovered that Rockey was less than honest about too many things to overlook. He wasn't a straight-up lie-to-your-face guy, but he was clever with omissions and diversions. Leaving my name off the deed to the farm is a fine example. When I asked him about it, he said he just forgot. He said he would fix it. He didn't forget, he never fixed it, and I'm sure he did it with intent to protect his investment. That incident seriously damaged my trust for him. Tossing me into a wall took another huge bite out of the trust I had for him. It also made me mistrust my own judgement. How could I have ended up loving a guy who would do that? What signs did I miss along the way that were shrouded in love? I was still sure he didn't mean it, but how badly had his brain been scrambled that he could do it now? I was disappointed in myself for returning to that house, his house. So, the air around us remained bruised for a long time.

I had been sleeping on the couch most nights for years. The couch-sleeping had started because Rock was a magnificent snoring machine and the couch was closer than the downstairs bedroom. Many Parkinson's patients suffer from night terrors and Rockey often didn't awaken while they were happening and rarely remembered them. They started as only an occasional nightmare in which he might yell and thrash around. By this time, he had them most nights and they were loud, and his thrashing was violent; sometimes he got out of bed to fight. The typical subject of these terrifying dreams were intruders. Coming into our home, into his shop, into his boat, always meaning to do him harm, and he was always fighting them viciously. I always figured it was related to his loss of strength, his loss of ability to protect the ones he loved, the loss of his identity as the biggest and the strongest. One night he yelled out with perfect diction, "Shoot the fuckers! Shoot the fuckers!" and jumped out of bed and began rummaging in a drawer. I would never have touched him in the middle of one these battles lest he mistake me for an intruder, but I called out to him to wake up. I called louder and he stopped digging in the drawer and I asked, "What are you looking for?" He looked at me straight-faced, although likely still not fully awake, and said, "My pistol. Where the hell is my pistol?" I was out of bed and flying across the room stopping six feet or so away and I shouted as loud as I could, "Rockey Goertz, you need to wake up right now!" He finally did and asked what was going on. I told him he was having a nightmare, and he turned and crawled back into bed without another word. I grabbed my pillow and headed for a couch in a faraway room. He could always go right back to sleep, but I'd lay listening to my racing heart for hours.

The next day I asked if he remembered his dream. He kept eating his cereal and said, "Yeah. There were men on the roof of the RV, and they were trying to get in."

I asked, "Where were you?"

He said, "You were there too, and we were down some long trailhead access road with nobody else around." I asked him if he remembered what happened and he said, "No. I must have woken up." Then I told him about looking for his pistol and he had no recollection of that. A couple days later, when Nick stopped over, I

83

asked him to unload that .357 for me. It didn't have a safety and I knew it had a hair trigger and I wasn't going to touch it. I hid the bullets and put the gun in a different place. Nick thought it was a good idea too.

Weeks later, out of the blue, Rock came out of the bedroom and said, "What happened to my pistol?" I explained what we'd done, and he said, "Why?" I told him I thought he might shoot me when he was in the middle of a night terror. He looked at me with great indignance and said, "I would never do that. How could you think that?" I replayed the dream about the RV marauders, the screaming, the shouting and the search for his gun. "How can I be sure you won't think I'm one of the fuckers that needs killing, Rock? It's not like you're awake and making sound decisions." He harrumphed away and put his gun back in his underwear drawer. I was making dinner a few hours later and he came and sat on one of the counter stools. He looked at me with a serious face and said, "You're probably right. You should put this wherever you think is safe. Sorry I scared you." And he gently laid the big gun down and went back to watch TV.

That fall a Forest Service cabin came up for sale. Well, not just "a" Forest Service cabin, it was one we had tried to buy years earlier, up one of the best trailheads in the canyon. They were hard to score as they rarely changed hands and usually sold before anyone knew they were available. We got lucky when I called the woman who owned it right away. I didn't dicker on price and told her I'd meet her at Four Corners to give her a check; payment in full was less money than a used pickup. Because of the way it worked, there wasn't a title company or a deed, we were only buying the building and continuing a land lease with the Forest Service. The paperwork was simple, and we completed the transaction sitting on a bench outside a little café. Rockey had written the check out of one of his secret accounts that did not bear my name, but again I made sure both of our names were on the paperwork. She handed me the key and said, "Have fun!"

. . .

Rock and I were both thrilled, and we each packed a bag, threw in the sleeping bags, food, water, warm clothes and the dogs and drove up the canyon past Big Sky to our new little primitive place. It was 16' x 20' and had an electric range from about 1950, a sink with no water but a bucket underneath—there was no running water—and a decent wood stove. There was pencil writing on one of logs from people who had been there; the earliest date I found was 1917. The previous owners were related to the people in the nearest cabin, and we were supposed to use their outhouse. Neither of us were keen on that idea.

This was one of my favorite trailheads in the Gallatin Canyon, and I told Rock I wanted to go hiking and see what I could see out there. He was going to make a fire and poke around. The dogs and I took off joyfully down the familiar trail, me dreaming of all this easy access to wilderness and adventures on foot and on horseback. The best news was that there wasn't another soul around. We walked a few miles until we came to a special place called Cow Flats. Here in this pine grove on my first wilderness trip, Rock and I had stopped to rest the horses and I had taken some of the best pictures I ever took of Rockey. That was twenty years earlier, when we were young and strong, beautiful and in love. I sat under the tree that I had tied my good old horse Elwood to that day. I looked around and saw where Rockey had hidden from me and come up a rise with his long strides laughing as I called his name. That laugh was the photo and it hung in our house. I felt uncharacteristically sentimental in that moment, and tears welled when I realized he'd never walk up again like that. Hell, he'd probably never smile at me again like that. I stood and gathered up the dogs and tried to shake the sadness by soaking in the beauty of the cliffs and hills around me as we headed back to the little cabin.

We had some simple good camp food for supper and sat on the creaky old chairs that came with the place. I put on some music from my phone, and we started talking about what we would do to fix up the joint. The chinking was rotten and there was plenty of daylight coming through. We were pleasantly surprised at the lack of mouse sign. We decided I'd order new twin mattresses— XL for the tall boy—and Rock would just tear apart the ancient bunkbeds and it would create a bit more room. I would tear up the rotten linoleum, and we could lay a tongue-and-groove pine floor together. He wanted it rewired as it looked as if it might have last been updated in the 1940s. I'd find some cheap fixtures to replace the bare bulbs. After the hard, shitty, combative year we'd had, it felt a little like a big sigh to sit together and be on the same page, even if it was only on a little thing for a little while. We were good at doing houses together.

Most of that winter, the cabin was the project *du jour*. The small demolition parts were easy and went fast. Rockey was never going to regain his physical strength. The typical Parkinson's gait is more of a slow shuffle. Rockey looked like he was moving faster than he could manage, so it always seemed as though he was going to fall forward. He told me it only felt unstable when he tried to stop, so he always had something in mind to grab ahold of, like a counter or a chair. Sometimes he would try to practice walking, and he would head down the driveway using ski poles for balance. I would peer out the window and just hope he didn't faceplant on the blacktop because it looked like such a difficult kind of locomotion.

The road past the cabin was not plowed in the winter; we parked in the ranch parking lot and walked in about a third of a mile. We put any supplies we needed in a big black plastic sled and pulled it in. The ranch used snowmobiles to pack the trail for sleigh rides, and somehow Rock moved with relative ease down this smooth snowy trail. Once we got all the things torn out that needed removal, Rockey started the chinking project. It isn't a very difficult thing to do, but it goes slowly, and our hands got sore. I helped a few days, but he liked going there alone. We both knew the manager from the nearby ranch, Marce, and I stopped to visit him one day on my way out to the cabin. He asked about Rockey's health, and I explained some and then let Marce know that Rock would be walking in some days to work on the cabin and maybe keep an eye on him. He said he surely would. By late winter, we had most of the interior chinked and Rockey was cleaning up for the day when he heard a snowmobile pull up just around sunset. He stuck his head out the door and greeted the rider, recognizing the ranch-owned sled.

The young man asked Rock if he was heading out soon.

Rockey replied, "Yeah, I'm just cleaning up my tools and will leave in a bit. Why?"

The kid smiled and said, "There's an elk been killed by a wolf just off the trail as you walk out. A big boar grizzly has been coming in every night to feed on the carcass and me and Marce didn't want you to end up being his dessert. So, I came to give you a ride back to your truck."

Touched by the thoughtfulness, Rock said, "Gimme two minutes and I'll take that ride."

Just as they passed by the opening where the carcass lay, they saw the big bear lumbering toward it through the timber in the dim light of the setting sun. When Rock got off at his truck, he clapped the young ranch hand on the shoulder and said, "Tell your boss thanks for looking out for this slow old man."

We were able to get a pickup back to the cabin by early April and we hauled in the pine flooring. Rock and I got it laid in two days, swept and cleaned the floor and threw on a coat of poly and went back home while it dried. He was noticeably uncomfortable after those two days of working on his hands and knees and I asked him what hurt. He said, "My back is messed up and it's not like the usual pain." Old concrete guys and construction workers are notoriously wounded fellows and Rock was no exception. He had several chronic lower back issues that had caused him pain for as long as I had known him. "What's different about it?" I asked.

"I don't know how to tell you. It's higher in my back and it feels like a tear maybe. It's a sharp pain, but it comes and goes. I'll get an appointment for a massage, that will help," he said. Rock let it drop and I didn't think much more about it at the time.

. . .

Spring was busy at the farm and a few early dry days let us get after a few things sooner than some years. The elk were hard on our fences over the winter when they broke in to eat the horse's hay, so we made a day of splicing breaks and replacing horseshoe nails that had popped off. I hooked up a short six-foot-wide section of the harrow and dragged a few horse pastures using the ATV, round and round for hours listening to music and singing loudly. Rock was disking a raggedy edge of the alfalfa field trying to add another fifty feet to harvest. Somehow, I got to thinking about the farm not having my name on it and I had just busted my ass for a few days making improvements to his place. That night after supper I asked him if he had ever gone down to the courthouse to add my name to the deed. He glared at me and said, "Why the hell do you care so much? It's yours anyway if I die because you forced me to marry you."

"What do you mean I forced you? I sure wasn't pregnant at forty-eight, so how is it that I forced you?"

"You were going to buy that land by Red Lodge and leave me. I had to marry you."

"I was going to buy a bare twenty-acre piece of land because I had the money, and I didn't own anything of my own. Why did you think I was leaving?" I asked incredulously.

He was getting madder, and I might have done better to try to deescalate things, but that was not what I did. I said, "It matters because you don't see me as a partner. It matters because that's what I thought this was about, being partners."

He stood up from his stool and yelled, "You've never done anything! I do everything and everything here is mine. It was all my money and all my work. Everything we have is mine."

This would have been the time for me to stop talking. I don't remember what I said but he stood quickly from his stool and grabbed my arm as I walked by and spun me to face him. In that moment he drew back that giant right hand and made a fist and a growling sound with the meanest look. I stared at the fist and thought of my mom and how sad she'd be for me to be staring down the same thing she had stared at. Then I shouted, "NO!" and yanked my skinny little forearm out of his grasp by dropping down. I spun and walked quickly out the door. This time I didn't run. I sat down on the steps, rubbing my arm and wondering why the fuck I was still here. This time he didn't apologize, but said, "Well you provoked me, didn't you?" when he found me crying on the steps.

I don't know why I didn't leave except that I was afraid. I was afraid he'd make it so I really would have nothing. And I'd have nowhere to go and no place to be. I cursed myself for allowing this to be my circumstance. I cursed him for being such an asshole. He went to bed on his end of the house, and I lay awake on the farthest away couch I could find.

In the morning, Rock walked out of the bedroom with a bag and said, "I'm going to work on the cabin for a few days." Then he was gone. I was glad.

I thought about leaving. All day. I thought about what money I had. I went to the bank and took another $2,000 out of our only joint account. I called two friends at opposite ends of the state from me: Marina, ninety miles south, and Laurie, about sixty miles north. I wanted them because Rockey didn't know either and could never find me. I drifted around the yard and house, unable to light anywhere. I thought how I would be vilified in my little community for walking out on that nice guy with all the health problems. I made a list called "The Years of Doing Nothing" showing hours and cost for the services I had provided in all those years of doing nothing. Laundry, cooking, landscaping, fencing, livestock management, medical management, mowing and on and on. I laughed out loud when I saw how much a person would spend to have all those things done for them. I knew he didn't value them at all.

It was a beautiful spring evening, and I was out walking with the dogs and about 10:00 p.m. I heard a banging in the horse barn and hurried, wearing my slippers, to investigate. My pal, my favorite Lenny, was cast with his head stuck under a gate and flailing to free himself. In the hours and days that followed that discovery, I learned that Lenny had colicked. In the middle of that night, I drove him to an equine surgery clinic about an hour away. They performed the surgery, did their best, and sweet Lenny died three days later. I was a pile of weeping horse girl in the aftermath.

Lenny was that horse that everyone who keeps horses hopes they get someday. The bond between us was nearly instantaneous and we took good care of each other. I never asked him to go anywhere that would hurt him and he never gave me a reason to be afraid. He was willing and seemed to thrive on our adventures, and we had so damn many. He was the one who returned the joy of riding to me, doused my fears, and made me laugh, he was such a clown. Losing him so young wrecked all my plans of us growing old together. I cried for months and am crying as I write this many years later. I was lucky to have been so loved by Lenny. I was lucky to have loved him so.

Big Drugs and No Relief

Rockey came home that evening. He was appropriately sympathetic, but of course that was little comfort. There wasn't much to talk about for a few days in the wake of our near miss with violence and the heavy sadness I felt. I suppose life just quietly drifted back into place, each of us keeping ourselves from the other, living in that bruised air again.

The pain Rock had been experiencing in his back grew in intensity and never really left. He saw a chiropractor, had acupuncture, more massages and even tried a few nights of a prescription muscle relaxer, but nothing offered any real relief. It was becoming worrisome because the pain wasn't like anything he had experienced before, and he had years of back pain. Rockey had always been hard-pressed to describe pain accurately or clearly. This thing in his back was six inches higher than his ruptured discs and he said it felt prickly, instead of the dull ache in his history. The way he had operated through years of chronic back pain was to just keep working.

He had gotten approval from the Forest Service on his own septic design for the cabin—no small feat—and was still going up there most days. Buffalo Creek ran in a curve around the cabin, so designing and constructing a septic system without disturbing this fragile creek was crucial to him and the success of this project. The land area was small, and every piece of equipment needed to have a spotter on the ground to assure proper distance from any water. I don't think it was physically taxing for him, but the constant pain was making him fractious.

Nick rarely discussed his dad with me, but during this time he asked, "What's going on with Dad? The job is going great but he's just so mad all the time." I said, "He's been having a rough time with his back and can't seem to get the pain under control." Nick replied, "It must be pretty bad, because his back has hurt every day of his life." I told him I had made some doctors' appointments for the next week and maybe he could get some answers.

The first appointment was with his primary physician, and he had no ideas and suggested Rockey see a back specialist. Coincidentally, that appointment was scheduled for the next day at an orthopedic clinic in Bozeman. We were both disappointed when an assistant to a different doctor at the Ortho place met us.

"You have to follow protocol before you can actually see the spine doctor," she said.

"Well let's get that going as soon as we can," Rockey said. "What do I have to do?"

"You'll need a scan with dye in your spinal column so we can detect where the problem might be." She suggested three weeks from that day.

Rock said, "Oh no. I can't wait that long. Why is it so far out? I'm in serious pain."

His words came out slow, a bit garbled and in a very soft voice, and I thought I recognized her impatience with Rock. She seemed to kind of give him the stink eye and said, "Fine, we can do it Thursday, but you can't have any sedation."

Rockey replied, "Well, I sure do think I'd need something for the pain before you stick needles in my spine, but if you think that's going work … okay."

We looked at each other, wondering why no sedation on Thursday, and Rock gave the head jerk toward the woman, so I said, "Why can he have sedation in three weeks, but not on Thursday?"

"That's just how we do it. Take it or leave it." I nodded sagely, not wanting to be the one to pick a fight and ruin his chances.

The woman left us in the room, closed the door, and Rock said, "Wow. She sure had the ass for me."

"Yup," I said. "I think you pissed her off right away. Just by being you. Now what?"

"Well, how bad can it be? I had brain surgery without sedation."

"It's your call, Rockey."

"I'm saying yes," he said.

The woman came back shortly with some papers and said Thursday at 1:00 p.m. This was surely one of the weirdest appointments Rock had experienced.

By the time of this appointment, his pain was much more severe. They gave him no sedation or pain medication, despite Rockey's request for one or both. They showed us to a small patient room, and someone came to get Rock for the scan while I stayed in the room. Not much time had gone by when I heard Rockey scream loud enough to carry through doors and down a hallway. I ran out the door and down the hall to a closed door where I heard the doctor say, "Whose idea was it to not have this patient sedated?" Then I heard Rockey say, "Just stop. Please just stop."

The door opened and a nurse came out, and I asked, "Are they done?" She rolled her eyes and nodded, hurrying away. When the door opened again, Rock was ashen faced being pushed in a wheelchair. I stuck my hand out to stop it and bent down asking, "Are you okay?"

He nodded and said, "Get me out of here."

I stepped into the handles, nudging the driver out of way, and started toward the door. I turned and said, "I want a CD of his records."

The nurse said "Sure. Stop in in a couple days. Do you want to schedule his next appointment?"

"No, he doesn't want another appointment and I'll be back in ten minutes to pick up those records."

Her eyes got wide, and she scurried off. I wheeled Rock out to my truck, and he was obviously in more pain than when we arrived. I asked what happened and he told me in a very whispery voice that they couldn't get the needle with the dye into his spinal cord because it's so swollen.

"So, what did they do?" I asked.

He closed his eyes and shook his head and said, "I think they just pushed harder. It was so bad, I nearly passed out."

I helped him into the truck and got him buckled in, reclined the seat a bit for him, rolled down the windows and ran back to get the records. The woman was coming out with an envelope in her hand. I snatched it from her, said thanks and turned back to get Rockey home. On the way home, I left a message for his primary doctor, requesting a prescription for some serious pain meds. At home, he stripped and got into bed while I rummaged around and found a bottle of Hydrocodone he'd had for his knee surgery. I gave him two, closed the door and started making phone calls.

It was time to give up on finding answers in Bozeman. Time for the big guns: Billings Neurology doctors. After several failed attempts to speak to a person and leaving messages, I remembered getting a direct number from one doctor's assistant who said, "Here's my direct phone. If you're not getting what you need, call me." I did and she answered. I went through the whole story from the beginnings of the pain months ago. She asked a few questions and said she'd get back me.

In the middle of these phone calls, I returned a missed call from the veterinary clinic. There were some lingering questions about Lenny's remains and Kimber had left a package there for me. I said I'd be there tomorrow and to please have the bill ready.

The pharmacy in Bozeman texted and said they had a prescription ready for Rockey from his primary doctor. I went into the bedroom and whispered to Rock that I was running to pick up that prescription, kissed his forehead and said I'd be back in an hour. I loaded up the dogs and took off.

On the drive, the assistant to the neurology doctors called back and said that she could get Rockey in for a cortisone shot in his spine on Tuesday. I reminded her that they were unable to shoot the dye in for the imaging because of swelling and she responded, "We will sedate him and numb the area." I asked why he had to endure the cortisone shot before getting an image. Her answer was, "Insurance requires us to try another method before doing expensive imaging."

"Okay, we'll be there," I told her.

Rock was still sleeping when I got back from town, so I ran down to the barn to quickly do the chores before starting dinner. The remnants of Lenny's last night there were something I still needed to clean up or at least bend the gate back into shape where he had been stuck. Tomorrow, I told myself as I hurried back to the house.

Rockey was awake, sitting in the living room watching the news. I got him some ice water, an ice pack and told him all the latest about the appointment in Billings and that the prescription I picked up was Dilaudid. I started grilling some chicken and making a salad. It was uncomfortable for Rock to sit at the table or the counter, so we ate in our big chairs in front of the TV. He thought the attempt to inject the dye had made something very angry in his back and had some reservations about the cortisone shot. I told him about the insurance requirement and said, "I'm not sure there's much you can do except let them try. It sounds to me like they won't go forward without this step."

The big drugs did their job, and he had a good night's sleep. He headed back to the cabin to continue the work on the septic, planning to get through the day with ibuprofen. I texted Nick and told him to try to keep Rock from picking up a shovel or a rake and maybe put a chair outside for him. He could still boss people around from a sitting position, I thought. I drove out to the vet clinic to pay my big bill and was given a beautifully wrapped package as I walked out. I opened it when I got in the truck, and it was a thick and complicated braid of Lenny's pristine white tail with a lovely note from Kimber. I turned it over with delicate hand movements, marveled at the artistry, felt grateful for the kindness and, of course, began this day with new tears.

Being alone for the day, I took advantage of the time and used my girl-sized, six-pound maul and a length of 2x4 to bend the gate back into shape. With my energy still low, it was a good day to ride around on the lawnmower and listen to music.

We ate sitting in our big chairs again, and I asked how the cabin project was going. He was pleased that the tiny bridge on the very bad road to the cabin had held the concrete truck, and they poured a slab to set the bathhouse on a few days ago. Rockey and some pals had built the small building that would be the bathhouse in the shop at our place in Gateway. On this day, Nick had loaded the little hut on a lowboy trailer and driven it up the canyon to be set on the slab. Part of the agreement with the Forest Service on the septic/bathhouse project was that we seed all disturbed areas with pre-approved native grass mix. Rock asked if I was ready for that step and I said, "Yup. I went to Cashman's and bought the seed mix the Forest Service approved and I can start anytime. I thought I'd bring that little submersible pump we have so I can sprinkle it. It's going to need a lot of moisture to germinate. We should water it every day for a few weeks at least. I think I'll haul those portable corrals up there too, so it will be ready when we can ride." Rock answered, "None of the ground was touched under those trees, so that part where you want to set up the corrals doesn't need seeding." We talked more about the work, and it was an easy conversation. He had always been comfortable, even in the worst times, talking about his projects. It was a relief to not have the air between us so charged and unhappy.

I spent long hours those days working on the gardens, both vegetable and flower. In some foolish time long gone, I had assumed I would always love the gardening thing and designed and planted way too many gardens. The perimeter of the yard had a rock border, which I had hauled and placed every rock for and planted with wildflowers and perennials. There were two big perennial gardens, two vegetable plots and container plants everywhere. And weeds. Plenty of weeds. As the years crept by and the challenges of caring for a person with a progressive disease became more time consuming, I kind of grew to hate the gardens and the work they required. But I had planted too much pride in with the flowers and food to let them go. Rock continued to go to the cabin most days and seemed to be wearing thin from the constant pain. He didn't talk much about it, but it was visible on his face in the pinches and the lines he carried. The prescription pain meds helped, but he was unwilling to take them during the day and only used them at night.

Tuesday came and we set off for Billings. He had an appointment to see Dr. Echeverri before the cortisone injection. The doctor expressed concern over Rockey's appearance, some weight loss, his lurching gait, the pinched face and the anguished eyes. He asked how long Rock had been experiencing this pain and I said, "Maybe a month or month and a half."

"Does anything help with the pain?" he asked.

I told him what Rockey had been prescribed and how he was using it and Echeverri asked him, "Why aren't you taking it during the day?"

Rock answered, "So I can work."

The doctor looked at me and rolled his eyes, and I said, "Yup,

97

that's our boy. You can't be surprised," and tapped Rockey's fore-head lightly and said, "Use your head, Rockne. Work less, rest more. You look rough. You might not be Superman."

We all laughed. He then explained that if the cortisone shot worked, he would get two more injections, two weeks apart. If it didn't offer any relief, they could push for the Myelogram, another kind of spinal imaging that used an injection of dye into the spinal canal. He gave us directions to the nearby surgery center and off we went to get his cortisone injection. I asked him to call in anoth-er pain medication for Rock before we walked away.

Rock was numbed up adequately in the area of the injection, so the pain wasn't excruciating like the last attempt. The doctor told me he was unable inject the full amount because of the swelling, and he would report that to Echeverri. It didn't work and instead of offering relief, his pain increased significantly. I called Echeverri's office a few days later to let him know, and they said he would go forward with getting Rockey an appointment for the Myelogram.

Haying season was upon us and Rockey was in no shape to do it. I called his friend and our good neighbor Bob to ask for help and he said he'd try to round some up.

I was gone for the day and when I arrived home, there were still a handful of guys in the fields moving bales with tractors and bobcats. I found Rockey sitting on the front porch glowering. I popped out of my truck with a big smile and said, "Wow! Pretty productive crew you've got here."

He wasted no time setting me straight. "Look at that field, it's a mess. There are wisps of hay everywhere that they missed with the baler. It looks like shit and I'm so mad, I even yelled at Wayne."

I looked out and yeah, there were some missed pickups of hay, but it certainly wasn't enough to be worth that attitude. I sat down in a porch chair trying to get a read on his sour face. I asked him how his pain was and whether he was taking his pain meds.

He glared at me and said, "The pain is terrible, and I am taking the pain meds, which is why I'm sitting on the porch. I can hardly walk, and I could never get up into the tractor, let alone run the baler. And yes, I'm taking the pain meds and they make me really crabby." More sentences than he had used in some time made me think I should proceed with caution.

"I'm going to start some dinner." The dogs came running for some hugs and I gladly doled them out. It didn't look like Rockey had eaten any of the food I left for him, but I started something fresh anyway. I heard him take off in the ATV and saw him drive down to the shop where the hay helpers had cracked a beer.

While we ate dinner, he remarked that Wayne had needed to take some small bales to feed his horses until his hay was ready. Then he added something I didn't hear, and I asked him to repeat it. He did and it was something about how much he charged him for the hay.

"Seriously? You charged Wayne for hay after he just spent two days doing your hay because you're wrecked and he's a nice guy?"

"Well yeah, we always pay each other for hay," he said.

I decided I was tired of being on the receiving end of his anger so held my tongue and took my half-finished plate of food to the kitchen. I went back in the living room a minute later and took his plate and glass from him and as I walked away, he said, "You don't like that?"

"I wouldn't have charged him. Your hay would still be in the field waiting on that big storm that's brewing if he hadn't come over. You yelled at him, and you charged him. No, I don't think I'd handle it that way. But it's already done, so it doesn't much matter what I think about it." I walked to the door and said over my shoulder, "I gotta go do some chores. I'll be back."

I knew his pain was great and his history with pain meds included an angry disposition with prolonged use. I felt bad that he was so thoughtless to our kind neighbors, but didn't see any way to mend it, because it wasn't my mess. I was thinking about how many doctor visits he already had under his belt with this intense and unnamed pain with no answers in sight and the toll it was taking on him. He looked bad. His face was drawn and carried new creases. Walking looked hard and almost dangerous, with a bad lean to the left. The near future looked grim.

I was sleeping on the couch when I heard him call out in the middle of the night. I hurried to him, and he was panting, groaning and moving his legs. He threw back the covers and said, "Look at this! I can't make it stop." The quad muscles as well as the muscles in his calves were spasming so hard and relentlessly, it looked like something alive under his skin. His feet were so cramped they bent downward.

I said, "Jesus, Rock!" and I started to try to rub the spasms out. It did no good and they just kept moving under my hands. I went digging through a drawer trying to remember what drug he might have for spasms and found some Flexeril. I dumped two onto my hand and set the tiny pills on his tongue and grabbed some water. Trying to think of a more immediate remedy, I said, "How about getting in the hot tub? Maybe the jets will help."

He stood and fell back onto the bed and said breathlessly, "I can't."

I ran and opened the tub, pulled him up by his arms and said, "Get ahold of my shoulders, I'll get you there and get you in." We made an awkward stumbling approach toward the tub on the deck.

"Now what?" he said.

I told him to sit on the edge and hold onto me again. He sat and I lifted and swung his legs over the edge and got in behind him with my pants on and helped him get seated and turned on the jets. I said, "Don't drown. I'm going to google this. Stay as long as you can stand it. I'll be right back."

The Mayo Clinic site said magnesium and potassium for spasms. I peeled a banana, gave it to him and went drawer digging for some magnesium, thinking he'd been taking it at some point for the spasms that sometimes accompany Parkinson's. His face indicated extreme pain and I hoped the Flexeril kicked in because I lacked faith in the banana to fix it. After I found the magnesium and gave him a couple, I sat by the edge of the tub and ran my fingers gently over his neck and shoulders, hoping to bring some relaxation to an unaffected part of his body. Even his upper body was rigid as he braced against the spasms. The caresses probably did no good, but maybe it offered some comfort to not be alone in this sudden onslaught by his own body. More times than I can count, that was all I could offer.

Getting him out of the tub was easier for him but almost knocked me over as he fell hard against me when he got both legs out. I held him hard around his torso and half dragged him back to the bed where he just fell into it. I picked up his legs and tried to straighten them and dragged some covers up and he screamed, "No! They weigh too much."

"Okay, okay," I said. "How about just the sheet?" He nodded.

He was breathless from the exertion and probably from the pain. I lifted the sheet and looked at his legs and the spasms were not as visible as they had been. I put my hands on his chest and asked him to lay back and try to take some deep breaths. He had never really been able to do that since that awful mule wreck and he didn't do it now. I said, "How about just trying to breathe slower? Slow inhale. Slow exhale." That worked better and I could see his face relax a little as I ran my hands gently over his chest and tried to slow my own breathing. It had been about forty-five minutes since he had taken the Flexeril, and it was beginning to quiet his legs, but not completely. I stayed by him and continued the slow motion on his chest. After a bit I asked if he thought he might sleep. He asked for the other pain pills, and I gave them to him. He said he thought he'd be all right and I told him I wasn't far away, and I left him to rest.

I found a notebook and wrote down the date and time and described what had happened and all the drugs I had given him. By the time this whole thing was over weeks from now, I would fill pages and pages with notes like these about events and all the drugs dispensed. I sat up with my legs stretched out on the couch, staring out the window at the moonlit fields and smoked every Kool cigarette he had. Except for one.

As soon as the clock hit 7:00 a.m., I dialed the neurology office. I left a message with Dr. Echeverri's assistant describing the events of the night before. By 8:00 a.m., I had a return call saying the doctor was going to change the meds and prescribe oxycodone for pain and Valium for the spasms. They told me how to stagger the dosing to get the maximum effect. I was able to get Rock to eat some toast and made sure he had ice water while I waited for the pharmacy to text that the prescriptions were ready. He said he wanted to move from the bed to his big chair, and I stood by as he tried to stand. He managed to stand, but was unable to take steps on his own, so once again I grabbed him hard around his torso as he leaned across my shoulders and I kind of pulled him along to the chair. Our height difference was working against me as his 6'3" frame draped over my 5'4", plus his seventy-pound advantage didn't feel much like an advantage to either one of us. I didn't dare think about what a shower was going to look like.

The pharmacy text came at about 10:30 a.m., just after I had given Rockey another Flexeril and Dilaudid. I told him I had to run to town for about an hour and asked what he needed before I left. He asked for help to the bathroom, so we did the drag/carry thing again and I got him back to the chair. I made sure he had his phone and asked him to please stay put. He smiled weakly at me and said, "I think I'm pretty stuck without my ride."

The act of showering was indeed a monumental task. He would kind of piggy-back on my shoulders and I trudged him to the edge of the shower. He would then grab the frame around the glass door and hold on while I lifted his legs over the two-inch lip of the shower. I had put a chair in the shower and would squeeze past him hanging onto the frame to once again have him lean on me as he lowered onto the chair. I would strip off my clothes, get in and use the shower wand to wet, soap and rinse him. He would wobble to a crouch leaning on my back to wash his nether parts and then I'd rinse him. He would stay seated in the chair while I dried the parts I could reach and then use my back to stand again and repeat the entry process in reverse. He was so exhausted after a shower I would lower him right into bed for a while. Daily showers became a distant memory.

Spiders

We lived like this for about two weeks until he was scheduled for the Myelogram. This was just an imaging appointment, so we didn't need bags, and the dogs rode in the back on the trip to Billings. At the St. Vincent's entrance, I parked and ran in to retrieve a wheel-chair while he waited. We made our way to the second-floor surgical center and got him registered. He was plenty drugged and still quite uncomfortable. The new drug regimen helped, but he hadn't been pain-free for weeks and was greatly diminished because of it. He looked haggard and thin with heavy-lidded, slow eyes. His speech was particularly affected by the drugs, which made him even more difficult to understand. The drugs had also made him sleepy, but when he was alert, he had that edge of nastiness that he had shown early in this opioid expedition and some nasty words came out as we waited to be called. It wasn't loud, but he was bitching at me about the wait, as if I had any control over it. I had been guarding and caring for him 24/7 for weeks now and rather than respond, I just moved across the waiting room knowing he would never create a public spectacle. I enjoyed my moments not sitting next to him, even if the move was petty. I was tired of running this show.

They finally called his name, and I wheeled him behind a nurse back to a surgical prep area, where the medical staff pushed him into a room. They helped him into a gown, then the bed, where they started an IV. He would be under general anesthesia for the Myelogram. He was so addled by the drugs, the pain and the length of the time leading up to this moment, he began to cry because he didn't know why he was there. I stroked his hair and explained the procedure again, and just then Dr. Goodman appeared. He was kind and patient and assured Rockey that he would find some answers. He told me Rock would be out in about an hour and he would find me in the waiting room. Just like all the other hospital adventures, once freed I bolted past the flock of blue chairs, down the stairs and into the fresh air outside. I took the dogs for walk in the hot city air. They were finally becoming more accustomed to sights and sounds of a more peopled setting. We took our time before heading back to the truck, where I put on some music and the air conditioning for the endlessly patient pups.

I had been sitting in a blue chair for twenty minutes longer than an hour when I saw a tall man come out of a room far down a hallway. I was the only one left in the waiting room, so I guessed the tall guy in the scrubs was coming for me.

He stopped and asked, "Are you Maggie?"

"Yes," I said. He stood in front of me and told me how difficult it had been to insert the needle with the dye into Rockey's spinal canal. I said, "Wait a minute, who are you?"

"I'm the radiologist," he said. He went on, and all I can remember is some derivative of the word arachnid. He told me they would take Rockey to recovery and someone would come and find me.

I went back to my book, and suddenly Dr. G came striding across the skyway. As he went by, he casually said, "I guess they didn't find anything."

"The radiologist just came out here and said something about spiders," I said.

He stopped abruptly and said, "What?"

105

I stammered and said, "Well, I don't know. He said a word that sounded like arachnid, and I don't know what that means."

"I've got to catch him before he leaves," he said, and he ran down the hallway. His reaction alarmed me, but there was nobody to ask, so I just sat and waited.

Eventually, Dr. G came back to the waiting room and his slow gait and posture told me the news would not be good. He sat next to me and said quietly, "Rockne has arachnoiditis. It's a chronic inflammation of the nerves in the spinal column."

I stared, thought for a moment, then said, "What does that mean for him?"

He sat back and for the first time didn't look like he was going to walk away, and he started to talk. He told me arachnoiditis was rare and incredibly painful. He said other patients had described it like being burned every minute. Because the inflammation was in the nerves, the pain was not localized and traveled everywhere. The doctor went on to say that as it progressed it impacted the nerves to the legs; that was why Rock was having so much trouble making his legs work, and this disease was the cause of the painful rolling muscle spasms he was experiencing.

"Does it go away or get better?" I asked.

He looked down and answered, "No, it doesn't go away and it's progressive. It doesn't get better."

I felt my chest constrict and asked, "How do you treat it? Is there a surgery for it?"

"There is no treatment. Surgery is ineffective and only causes bleeding and does nothing to remedy the source of the problem."

"Well, how do people live with it then?"

"They don't," he said. "The pain is so horrific most people can't live with that kind of pain."

"So, they kill themselves?" I asked.

"That or they experience a psychotic break. But we can install an intrathecal pain pump." He stood up and touched his abdomen and said, "We install the reservoir here. The reservoir is about this big," and he cupped one hand, "and we run a small tube around his side, and it runs through a tiny battery in his lower back." He turned and pointed out the placement of the battery. "Then the catheter continues up his spine and will end above the point of inflammation. We fill the reservoir with some combination of narcotics, and as the pump pushes the liquid up the tube, it will bathe the inflamed area to numb the pain. This method allows us to use a fraction of the dose, about 1/300th, required to control the pain with oral medications and therefore causes less side effects. Because of the tiny dosing, his mental capacity will remain unaffected as well."

I sighed and shook my head. "Will he see a return of the function in his legs?"

The doctor said, "Probably some, but you know Parkinson's continues to affect his mobility and any stretch of time like this where he is immobile is likely to be difficult to completely recover from. It will depend on how hard he's willing to try. He will be quite weakened by the time the pain recedes. How long has this been going on?"

"He's been in real trouble for three weeks but has been taking pretty big pain meds for six. How long does the reservoir last and how do they fill it? Please tell me it's not another surgery every time."

He smiled a faint smile and said, "No, not surgery. There is a port at the top of the reservoir, and the pain doctor will use a needle to extract any remaining liquid at his refill appointment and then refill the reservoir with new drugs. The longevity depends on the volume of the dosing drip. The pain clinic will calculate when the patient needs a refill and book his next appointment when he leaves. The average refill time is four to six months. It has a built-in alarm that sounds if the supply gets low."

"Where is this pain clinic and who is that doctor?"

"The pain clinic is in the building across the street and is run by

Dr. S," he told me. "I am a partner in the business end of it, but do not practice there. You need to understand that the drugs dispensed out of the pain clinic are often federally regulated Schedule 1 pharmaceuticals, and the pain clinic itself has federal oversight. It's a very no-nonsense place and I've heard him referred to as the drug Nazi. He's very tough. It's serious business to maintain licensing and it's run under very strict protocols. Dr. S can explain more and answer any questions when you meet with him."

"Well, I sure hope you're going to be the one to tell Rockey. This is pretty devastating, but at least there is a way out of the pain."

He held out his hand to help me up and said, "I know where he is. Let's go talk to him."

As we walked, Dr. G said, "We need to run a test to see if Rockne can handle the drugs we would put into the pump. Has he had any experience with morphine?" I answered yes and said that he tolerated it well. "I'd like to admit him tomorrow for an overnight stay and dose him with morphine to see how he does."

I said, "Why can't he just stay the night tonight?" He told me that because he was here for a day surgery, they can't admit him directly; there has to be a night in between for insurance to pay. Another big sigh from me. "So, we need to get a hotel tonight and then check back in here tomorrow?"

"Ideally. Can you do that?"

"Yes, but I can't stay two nights. Once he's settled tomorrow, I'll have to run home and take care of the horses and stuff and then come back the next day. Can he go home Thursday?"

"Yes, and we will schedule the surgery for the implant before he leaves."

"Just don't leave us in the lurch without access to more pain meds," I said. "He'll never make it without them. And please don't talk to me about addiction right now. He'll deal with that if he must when we are at the end of this. He's done harder things and he can do that too."

We found Rockey's room and once again I was struck by how haggard this once handsome guy looked. Deep circles under his eyes carrying deeper wrinkles in his face than just a month before. I thought to myself that pain was a wicked companion. I could also see the lingering effects of anesthesia as it took him a moment to recognize Dr. G. I leaned in, cupped his face, and kissed him softly, asking how he felt. "Groggy. Did you figure it out?" he said to the doctor.

Dr. G started to talk, and I backed away a little in the small space allowing him to be front and center. I didn't think Rock was grasping all the explanation, but I kept watching his face for a reaction. Parkinson's patients also experience a thing called masking, when their facial muscles no longer adequately display emotion which further impedes their ability to communicate. Often their words don't match their facial expression or lack of expression. His face was still as a stone, but I watched his eyes, looking for some kind of tell.

The doctor gave Rock a much-abbreviated explanation of the one he had shared with me about what he found and what it meant. He got to the end and stopped. We both waited for Rockey to speak. He looked at Dr G and said, "Okay. When do we operate and get this thing out of there?"

The doctor said, "No, Rockne. We can't take anything out. There is no cure and there is no treatment to make it go away." Rock was silent for a moment and repeated the same question, and Dr G looked at me, and I just raised my eyebrows and indicated that the stage was still his. He tried to explain again and Rockey just stared at him with icy eyes and said, "If you think I can live like this, you're nuts." The doctor pulled up the chair and sat down so he was at eye level with Rock and told him about the pain pump and all that went along with that. I was sure now that Rockey wasn't getting much of it; at the end he said, "Can I get it tomorrow?"

"No, it will be a few weeks, because it's awfully expensive and it has to be preapproved by your insurance company before we can schedule it."

Rock looked at me and back to the doctor and said, "Give it to her. She can make anybody do anything and do it right now."

I laughed and shook my head, and the doctor said, "We'll get it rolling right away. You have my word. Do you have any more questions?" Rockey turned away from him and faced the wall and gave no more acknowledgement to his presence. I walked a few steps away with Dr. G, and he said, "We'll release him as soon as his blood pressure goes back down. You should be out of here in a half hour. I'll have the nurse give you the orders for the morning and I'll see you then. Good luck tonight. Do you have the pain meds you need to get through the night?"

I said, "Yeah, we're good. See you in the morning." As he walked away, I turned to go back and sit by Rockey.

He flung back the covers and started to pull on his IV line and I grabbed his hand and said, "Hey, hey. What are you doing?"

"Get me the fuck out of here if they can't help me."

I spoke softly and said, "Just wait a minute now. They're getting another prescription for you and your blood pressure has to be normal before they let you out tonight. We'll get going pretty quick." I lied about the prescription. "We'll get to the hotel, and I'll order Chinese or pizza, what sounds good?"

He said as he laid his head back, "Chinese. I'm starving."

"Me too," I said. "Now just chill a little and we'll be eating in no time." I was now using child logic to calm my tormented husband.

When we checked into the hospital the next morning, we were told that Dr. S would be by to meet with both of us at 10:00 a.m., so I postponed my trip back to the farm to take care of the horses. They would be keeping Rockey overnight this time, so I planned to leave after that meeting and come back the next day to pick him up. For all his fierce reputation, I didn't find this doctor to be scary at all. He brought literature that he left with us and spent a long time talking quietly with us about the Medtronic pain pump, how it worked and how it would impact Rock's life. He was direct with me about my role as Rockey's caregiver, which didn't really change what I was already doing. After lots of talk, I took Rockey's hand and asked him if he had any questions. He said, "Yeah. When are we going to start this morphine test? This pain is eating me up and I haven't had any pain meds for hours. Can we get on with it, please?"

I said goodbye to Rock and Dr. S and told Rock we could talk later but I'd be back in the morning to pick him up. I tried not to think about the past two days or two months as I gassed up my truck, bought a pack of cigarettes and pulled out onto the freeway with the music cranked up, the windows down and the cruise set at 80 mph as soon as I could. I turned off my phone just past Laurel and settled in for a mindless drive home.

Psychotic Break

Leaving Rockey in the hospital for the morphine tolerance test at St Vincent's, I made it back to the farm by about 1:00 p.m., got the horses squared away and let both dogs run wild for a bit. My dream of a long shower came true, followed by a change into soft, baggy clothes and sitting in a chair on the front porch with a cup of fresh coffee. The hummingbirds were engaged in a miniature version of a feeding frenzy, doing their aggressive dive-bombing, and screeching at each other. Not for the first time, I thought if hummingbirds had teeth, there would be a blood bath the way they fought. I watched them and stared at the bright pink phlox and yellow daisies in my untended garden, feeling grateful to be sitting right there. All the information I had ingested in the past twenty-four hours flew around in my head like pinballs and I wasn't having much success processing any of it, but this was a great spot to settle my thoughts.

I brought my laptop out to do an internet search on arachnoiditis and found a paper from a study done by a medical student in the UK. On every site I tried, this same paper was the only source of information. The paper discussed the high level of intractable pain and mentioned a few of the symptoms Rockey was experiencing. The paper speculated on the causes being a traumatic fall, invasive back procedure, injections in or near the spinal column or a type of dye no longer used for imaging. I know for sure Rock had a long fall off some scaffolding and several types of injections near his spine. For me, the "why" didn't matter as much as how it would affect his future. The paper said it was progressive and degenerative but was unclear beyond that. It did say there was sometimes permanent nerve damage to a patient's legs, interfering with mobility.

Subsequent searches didn't turn up more information or studies. It seemed no one knew much about arachnoiditis.

I returned a text to my sister Kathy, who was somewhere in northern Wisconsin enjoying a sunny summer day by a lake. She had been my person to talk to during these weeks of searching for answers and knew what Rock was going through. I know she cried sitting by that lake when she googled the word on her phone. The outlook was bleak. I told her in text talk that he may get a pain pump, and all was not yet lost. "More details later, no crying by the lake." But her admission was all I needed to finally let my own tears fall. It seemed that the past four years had been one tough break after another for Rockey. He would work so hard and make some meager progress recovering from one event or surgery and be knocked back again with something more formidable. This thing, arachnoiditis, was most sinister because I could see the pain, but the murkiness of the information about the disease itself and the track it might take was disheartening.

Rockey called me at the dinner hour. His voice was very soft and difficult to hear, but he thought the morphine test was successful. He said, "No bad reaction and no pain for hours." I asked whether the doctor had scheduled the pain pump surgery, and he answered, "No, tomorrow when you're here." I told him I'd be there by 11:00 a.m., talk to the doctor and bring him home. He said, "Good," and said goodnight.

I put away my computer and tried to find a tiny slice of peace on this lovely summer night. The full moon was waning, but it cast a lovely light as I set out across the stubble on the hayfield with my dogs. I put aside, or at least I tried to, thoughts of diseases with weird names, pain and more drugs and fewer answers. I walked through the soft light and paid attention to the gentle breeze across my face and the silhouette of Noonmark, the half-burned mountain above the farm. It was the best thing I could think of to quiet my questions and soak up some goodness.

I arrived back at St. Vincent's just before 11:00 a.m. and found a man in excruciating pain. I tried to ask him what was going on, and when he had last been given any pain meds. "A long time ago. Oh god, it's so bad," Rock said through clenched teeth. I found a nurse and asked the same questions. His pain medication had been dispensed within the past ninety minutes, so he should have been feeling some relief. I asked her what he'd been given in the past twelve hours and the amounts of each dose and she asked me if I had any ideas about what was different now that his pain was breaking through the medications. I said, "Maybe the dye injection was irritating the inflamed nerves. Have you been giving him Valium? I don't see it on here." The nurse scrolled through some computer entries and said, "It looks like it's been dropped off." I asked if they could try that on top of the Oxy and she said there was no doctor's order for it. I asked her to try to get that on his chart and maybe try to reach the neurologist if Dr G was unavailable. I had his Valium with me, but I didn't think I should give it to him in case I was missing something in his recent history. I went back to Rockey's room and did what I could to help him get more comfortable. I helped him reposition to lay on his side with his legs drawn up, which only gave him relief for a few minutes.

I was shocked to find him in this condition. This level of pain was over the top and the escalation didn't make sense to me unless the dye injection was responsible. I went back to the nurses' station and asked again if the doctor had sent an order for more drugs. The answer was no. Rockey's pain created a discomfort in me that

I still find hard to describe. Maybe it's exactly what to expect when you find yourself unable to provide any comfort, any release, any relief to someone you love from this kind of pain trap. I found myself contorting with each grimace or moan. He had always been stoic about his daily aches and pains and to hear him uttering painful sounds heightened the anxiety of the situation. I rubbed my face, I held my belly, I held my breath and then sighed deeply. And I paced. Then paced some more in the small confines of his room. I tried to softly touch his shoulders, his chest. I stroked his hair. I went back to the nurses' station and found no joy. I started calling the doctors' offices myself and leaving more frantic messages each time.

Finally, just past noon, Dr. G and Dr. S came in. I stepped back so they could engage with their patient. They asked Rock some questions and quickly ordered more drugs for him, including re-issuing the order for Valium. I asked if they were willing to give him morphine again to help get his pain level back to something we could handle on our own. "I can't take him home if he's in this kind of pain. I have no way to manage this. You have to do something to get this pain backed off before he's released," I said. They had some doctor words back and forth and said they could keep him another day and try to quiet whatever had cut loose to create this new version of the nightmare. They also thought that the dye had probably irritated the already oversensitive nerve bundle but hoped with some heavy doses of an anti-inflammatory drug and stepped-up pain management, they could get the pain down to a level we could deal with at home. They agreed to administer morphine for one more day but would not send us home with any.

The conversation then turned to the schedule for implanting the pain pump. Once again, I found Rockey was at the mercy of the insurance company and how quickly they shuffled papers; the doctors said it would take three weeks. That seemed an interminable wait and Rockey groaned loudly and cursed softly. The doctors in charge of relief flanked his bed and reassured him that he could have whatever he needed to get through to this date of August 7, 2014.

115

I stayed around for the rest of the afternoon. I left to buy him a fancy coffee and some cookies and find some take-out food he might like. He did manage to eat some, and the coffee and cookies brought him a moment of pleasure. The morphine and the other pile of drugs had subdued the pain and his alertness. I had a long talk with the nurse who would be watching over him and asked politely to be sure he never fell behind on the drug schedule. As we made our way through this pain-filled chapter, I realized that everything went more smoothly if the drugs were administered on time. If we fell off the schedule and the pain took hold, it took much longer to get it calmed down again. I also asked her to alternate the drugs, so he could have that layering effect of the pain management. I sat on his bed and stroked his face softly. He had lost the tightness of the grimace and although he looked haggard, at least his face was relaxed. I told him I was heading home and that he was staying in the hospital again and luckily, he was too dopey to care. I wrote my cell number on the whiteboard in his room and left it at the nurses' station as well. I had a few hours of daylight left as I drove toward home into the setting sun.

I called Nick on the drive home to give him an update and told him I'd go back tomorrow to fetch his dad. I asked him to go to the local medical supply place and get Rock a wheelchair and bill it to me, so I could move him around the house a little easier. I called my sister Kathy, and she said all the right big sister things to soothe my aching heart. She offered to come stay with me and I said it was not necessary because I had no way to predict what the coming weeks might hold for us. I said, "Maybe he will just sleep until it's time for the surgery. I'll be ok, but thanks." Had I only known what the weeks ahead held in store.

Back to Billings in the morning and I had Rockey in my truck heading for home by mid-afternoon. The drugs they administered in the hospital had finally managed to cut the sharp edges off the pain, and he was not only sedated but looked almost comfortable as we hurtled down the highway toward to the farm. Nick was at the house when we arrived and helped get his dad up the three steps and settled into his bed. I asked him to stay with Rock for a while so I could run to town for groceries, prescriptions, and some medical supplies. I bought a walker with a seat and hand brakes hoping it would allow Rock a little more independence to move around the house without having to call for help. I parked in the garage and entered the house to find Rockey sleeping in his chair with no one around. Furious, I looked out the window and saw Nick's truck down at the shop. I decided to save that confrontation for another day but crossed him off my list as a source of help. There was no way that Rock should ever be left alone for more than a few minutes in his current state, sleeping or not.

I worked quietly to put the groceries away and get some dinner started, and when Rockey stirred, I got him some fresh ice water and sat down beside him to see how he was doing. The great drugs from the hospital were wearing off and he was due for another dose of Oxy and Vallum. I could see the look of pain creeping back into his face and watched as he twisted and turned, trying to find a comfortable way to be. The tightness in my gut was creeping back, wondering how the evening and night would progress. It felt as if I was waiting for a storm.

The storm broke a few hours later, and poor Rockey was besieged with more muscle spasms and searing pain in his back and legs. I looked at the calendar for the hundredth time, wondering how the fuck he could endure this for three more weeks. We had been trying to navigate this thing for nearly six weeks and now, maybe from knowing what it was, the pain was even more relentless than when we were searching for answers. Although I respected his doctors, I realized that this road leading up to the surgery was going to be one that we traveled mostly alone. Whether it was because the source of his pain had only the one extreme remedy or something else, there didn't seem to be much available to us in terms of answers or direction as to how to get from here to there. All we had were a few bottles of narcotics and a date on the calendar.

The drug administration log I kept was precise and detailed, showing not only the times and dosages, but how intense his pain was at many intervals throughout the day and how long he slept after each dose. That night I decided to shorten the window between each dose by a half hour, hoping to get a jump on the pain before it returned each time the meds wore off. I calculated carefully to make sure this didn't put Rockey over the maximum milligrams of either drug recommended in a twenty-four-hour period and was relieved to find we had more room to modify the schedule without overdosing him. I was pleased with my ingenuity and thought maybe we could get a leg up on this rotten ride he was on.

Any appearance of victories in this period was false and the illusion short-lived. I tried to keep a schedule of sorts for meals he barely ate, pestering him about drinking water, and the occasional wrestling match into the shower. Rockey had always been fastidious in his personal appearance and the thought of only occasional showers went against a lifetime of habits. The act of getting into and out of the shower was so horribly painful, he made a rough peace with this new schedule. He needed to drink lots of water because his liver was compromised, and it labored inefficiently to filter these heavy drugs, because the drugs themselves suppressed all digestive and endocrine activity in his body. He fought me about insisting that he drink water because it created more painful trips to the bathroom. "If I don't drink, I won't have to pee," was his rationale. While I wouldn't give in or stop pestering him, I didn't realize the small decreases he was making in his water consumption, and that would come back to terrorize us both.

More Pain

The weeks crept by. Days and nights ran together, sleep became elusive for both of us, and the level of anxiety in our house from Rockey's constant and growing pain was palpable. Brittle is a good word to describe his state of being. Everything was too much. The sun coming in through the windows was too hot, too bright. The clicking sound the dogs' toenails made on the wood floor was agitating to him and he yelled to me to put them outside. There was no place and no position for Rock to find comfort and he was mostly unable to even turn halfway over in bed without help from me. Sometimes, he needed to switch positions as often as every fifteen minutes. I was exhausted from the lack of sleep and the exertion of moving this big guy around over and over every day. I continued to increase the amounts and/or the frequency of his drugs, but it only made a noticeable difference for a day at a time. The only reason I left the house was to do the fifteen minutes of chores and even that made me feel like I needed to hurry back. I watched it, I heard it, I tried to diminish it and yet to this day, I cannot imagine what that level of pain did to Rockey every day for so many weeks with only the dream of that far-off date to provide any relief.

119

Three days before the scheduled surgery to install the pain pump, the doctor's office called to tell us it had been postponed and rescheduled for three weeks later, making it August 27. I am a big truth teller and have rarely had a second thought about giving someone the straight up facts. When the office called, I had unintentionally wandered outside with the phone. I pleaded and argued to keep the original date to no avail. I was surprised to find I wasn't sure how to tell Rockey the truth. His mental and emotional stability were so fragile, his mind becoming so cloudy and unclear because of the drugs, the pain, the exhaustion, I worried for his sanity.

When I told him, he was silent for several minutes. He stared straight ahead, and two fat tears streamed down his face. He slowly raised his eyes to mine and said, "I don't think I can make it, Mag. It's just too much." Then he asked, "How many days?"

I took in a big breath and whispered, "Twenty-three. It's twenty-three days."

"Fuck," was all he said.

When this waiting game began, Rock was firm in stating he didn't want to take the maximum amount of drugs he was allowed per day. He knew it would take a toll on his body and his mind, and he wanted to go through with the smallest amount needed to make the pain tolerable. That all changed the day they postponed the surgery. He said, "Fuck the moderation and give me all I am allowed to have, all day every day." I couldn't or wouldn't argue with him, and I referred to the drug log I had been keeping. The amounts he had been taking were significant, but still under the daily maximum allowed. The current level was not enough to ever knock him out completely and he rarely got any rest except to doze off now and then. He was mostly awake and mostly in agony. I wondered if upping the doses would finally let him get some real sleep. I couldn't blame him for throwing all caution to the wind.

Rockey's appetite was nearly non-existent and as the medications increased, his desire to eat decreased. I tried to fix a few things each day to entice him to eat but was mostly unsuccessful. His system became so sluggish from the drugs that constipation was an everyday problem. The act of walking to the bathroom was so painful I can only imagine what he went through in his mind to avoid it. I got him a portable urinal, but he found that difficult to use too.

As his condition continued to deteriorate, his pain levels increased, and real sleep was a distant memory. I camped out on the couch just outside his bedroom and felt lucky to catch an hour of uninterrupted sleep as Rockey got about the same. The edginess and anxiety in our house was monumental. Any peace was short-lived and being responsible for someone in such tremendous pain was beyond daunting. Even though I knew intellectually that I was giving him the best care, the best attempts at dulling his pain, I continually felt my efforts were inadequate and that I was not up to the task. I pestered the doctors with questions and found myself begging for answers or some secret form of relief that they might have forgotten. I paced the house wanting to join Rock in his vocalizations of pain. I developed a weird habit of rubbing my left eyebrow with such force, by the end of the summer, it had naked patches. My sister told me that when she talked to me on the phone, I no longer cried, but she could hear me holding my breath as I released those breaths in long sighs. Poor Rockey was endlessly miserable.

It was in the pacing one day, trying to think of anything I could do for him, that I remembered part of my conversation with Dr. G the day they diagnosed the arachnoiditis. The doctor had listed the things they believed might cause the disease.

"Any trauma to the back might create the perfect storm to form a pathway for it," he said. "A bad fall, repeated back injuries, a certain kind of dye used in scans, but no longer on the market, injections into the spine like a poorly placed cortisone shot."

I remember looking at the floor and shaking my head, saying, "Rockey had about a twenty-foot fall off some scaffolding ten years ago, he had a terrible mule wreck and broke nine ribs, he had some kind of radio frequency surgical procedure on his back in 1998, but there was no incision, and he's had multiple cortisone shots in his back for years, plus he was a concrete guy for twenty years, which puts enormous daily stress on a back." I stared off thinking and suddenly said, "And then there was the stem cell treatments."

Dr. G stood up and turned to look at me and asked, "What stem cell treatments?"

I proceeded to tell him about the stem cells, Russia, and the American company behind it. He asked for details about the procedure, and I explained, "They would remove about this much spinal fluid," indicating with my fingers. "And then they would inject a solution containing the stem cells about equivalent in volume into his spinal column."

"How many times?" he asked.

"Once a year for five years," I said. "The last one was in 2011." Dr. G was a quiet, reserved and kind man, but I was sure I saw anger flash in his eyes.

I offered to get in touch with the doctor from California who was present for the transplants and have him call Dr. G. He gave me his cell phone number and stalked away. I called Jay right then, and he said they had never had any complications like this, and he would be happy to call Rockey's surgeon. I know they talked, but neither of them ever told me what was said. Looking back on it now, I recall that Jay called a few times to check on Rockey, sent some supplements to aid in his digestive issues, but by summer's end, we never heard from him again. For a guy who had called a half dozen times a year for eight years, his absence was notable.

Untethering

August days seemed to creep by, and each one was filled with pain that Rockey seemed less and less able to endure. The helplessness I felt was bottomless as his moans and occasional screams cut though me, his clothes made a rustling sound as he turned, shifted in the chair or the bed, searching for some sweet spot where the pain didn't live. The sounds of desperation scraped at my heart. I looked at the drug log obsessively, watching the clock and waiting for the next dose of something. I made chocolate pudding, scrambled eggs, and a killer chicken and wild rice dish to spark his appetite, but nothing worked. I had this feeling of wanting to implode so I could stop holding my breath and leave this air full of angst and tension far behind. My body ached from lack of food, lack of sleep, buckets of coffee and days of holding tension in every limb while the only real remedy was twenty-some days away. I loved going to do the chores; the fifteen minutes away from the house and Rockey's pain brought me a sliver of relief. But my husband could find none.

Approaching mid-August, every day was the same. Rockey's face was lined with pain. He was breathless as he asked again and again for help switching positions. He had not yet reached the maximum dose allowed on either the oxycodone or Valium, and the Valium was starting to be less effective on the rolling spasms in his lower body. By Tuesday of that week, he seemed to be slipping away from reality. He imagined appointments we needed to keep and spoke often about dying.

"Do you think you can die from too much pain?" he asked more than once. I didn't tell him that the doctor had told me that some patients simply go insane.

He was beginning to float in and out of lucidity and still I didn't notice how drastically he had reduced his water consumption. He was so edgy from both the drugs and the pain, I tried my best to be invisible, to little avail because he needed my help for the simplest things. One evening, we were sitting in the living room in our big recliners and he pressed the button on his chair and sat straight up and said, "I know what to do."

"Do for what?" I asked.

"For the pain." He mumbled.

Here are the actual words I wrote in a journal that day:

Today his pain level remained high in the morning. After a painful and sleepless night, He had that wild-eyed look when I found him in his chair. I gave him one of each Oxy and Valium and by 9am he was sleeping in bed. I tried to keep his drug levels high for the day. For some continuous rest, the cost is confusion, loss of appetite, a brain so foggy he cannot make words. He put jeans and a Carhartt shirt on and headed off to put shoes on—sure we were going to see something. The silver lining in today was that his Valium prescription was refilled. 25 pills for 12 days.

These are the things he said:

"I'm allergic to canvas"

"maybe I should lay on the floor"

I think it's too hard & would hurt you...

"how about the vinyl?"

"Maybe the nylon"

nylon what?

"sleeping bag"

He turns steady for 45 minutes tonight. 3-5 minutes in each position. Sweaty with the effort. Needing more and more of my help with each change. Back, side, child's pose. ... Each one started fresh from a standing position beside the bed. Short, shallow gasping breaths. Not an ounce of comfort to be found.

Back out in the living room at midnight ... "spray me with glue."

This went on all night. My arms were covered with tiny red and purple marks, broken blood vessels from the strain of lifting him over and over. We were both completely, totally exhausted with not a moment's rest. Just before 6:00 a.m., I called his son Nick and said, "Your dad is in real trouble and we need to take him to the hospital." He said he could come right over; he lived just ten minutes away. I watched the clock and helped Rockey move from spot to spot seeking comfort, seeking some peace, talking nonsense all the while. By 7:00 a.m., Rock was nearly broken. I helped him lay down on the bed and called 911 for an ambulance, thinking Nick had just gone back to bed. As he lay on his side, he began to sob uncontrollably. I spooned behind him, holding him tight, crying and rocking gently, telling him softly that it would be all right.

That's how the EMTs found us when they came into the house with Nick trailing behind them. Nick lost it when he saw us and ran from the house in tears. I had to uncoil from the double fetal position we had worked ourselves into so I could talk to the EMTs. It was hard to be succinct in describing Rockey's condition with the weeks and layers it had taken for him to be in this shape. No one had ever heard of arachnoiditis and, really, it sounds like a made-up disease, so I talked about chronic inflammation in his spinal cord and heavy drugs while waiting for a pain pump. As they loaded my sobbing husband into the bus, I kissed his hand and told them I'd follow in my truck after I took a little time to explain to Nick what had been happening in the past week and his dad's steady decline as the pain grew stronger. The last time Nick had seen Rock, he was sitting in his chair, uncomfortable for sure, but crabby from pain and still talking sensibly. The dad he saw, curled up and weeping, shocked him badly, and while I felt perpetually disappointed in Nick's inability to step up and help his father more, I was keenly aware of and empathetic to his horror at the sight.

Nick took off ahead of me to be there when they transported Rockey into the ER in Bozeman. I needed to retrieve the bottles of meds he'd been taking and bring along the dosage log. No time for brushing teeth or hair or changing into clean clothes, I raced behind them on skinny backroads trying to be there for the inevitable questions.

When I walked in, there was a doctor by Rockey's bed trying to get answers. After weeks of drugs before and since his diagnosis, Rockey had absolutely no idea what was causing this pain and was damn mad about having to pee in a bottle. I closed the curtain for his privacy and walked the doctor a little way down the hall, leaving Nick to watch over his father. I gave the doctor a shortened version of the past two months, the increasing mystery pain, the many appointments with no diagnosis, increasing meds and finally the diagnosis and the waiting game for the pain pump installation.

"How long has he been altered?" he asked.

I told him, "I noticed it vaguely and only occasionally about a week ago, but he became completely unhinged in the past twenty-four hours." He asked if I thought he'd fallen or had a stroke; I answered no. He had never heard of arachnoiditis, and I said, "It's a chronic inflammation of the arachnoid. There is no cure and no treatment, and the only relief will be when he gets a pain pump, two weeks from now. You could google it." I showed him the bottles and my drug log and told him I thought that these weeks of heavy drugs had somehow become toxic in his system.

He looked through my notebook and said, "You're not giving him the max doses of any of these, why do you think that is?"

I said, "Rockey has always been sensitive to drugs and overreacts to lots of medicines. These may not be maximums, but isn't it a lot of drugs for six weeks for guy with a bad liver and a half dozen other things wrong? This altered state he's in has been gaining momentum. A week ago, he was just in a lot of pain and now he still has all the pain but seems to have fallen off the edge of reason. What else could it be? Can someone actually go insane from pain?"

He looked at me for what seemed a long time and shook his head. "I'm an ER doctor and I don't know what's going on with your husband. I'll examine him and check a few things out and we'll see what we can figure out. Okay?"

We walked back to see Rockey, who was talking loudly to a nurse and pointing at Nick, "He stole my truck so he can sell it for the money. He can't just do that, can he?" As I came through the curtain, he pointed at me and said, "She's in on it, too. They're trying to sell my farm and put me in a rest home. Don't let her fool you."

My first thought was that he was no longer doubled over in pain. I looked at Nick, who looked stricken, and gave my head a little shake. I took Rock's hand and he jerked it away with an angry glare. I said, "Rock, we didn't steal your truck and we can't steal the farm. We're here to try to figure out how to make you more comfortable. Remember, you're getting a pain pump put in to help with your back pain. Your truck is at home in the garage right where you left it."

His angry face lightened some and he asked, "Well, how did I get here then?"

I looked at Nick and he moved closer to the bed and said, "Dad, you came in an ambulance and Mag and I drove behind. We have to get some fluids into you, you're real dehydrated. Did you forget to drink your water?"

Rock's angry face came back, and he snapped, "No I didn't forget. It makes me have to pee." The doctor moved in, and I stepped back as he started to ask Rockey questions. Now it was Nick's turn to summon me with a head jerk and I followed him into the hall.

Nick asked, "What did you find out?"

"Nothing," I said. "They're going to try to figure out why he's so goofy. What about the dehydration?"

"They came in and said he was dehydrated, started an IV and catheterized him. His urine was so dark, it was almost brown."

"Oh geez. I haven't been paying close attention, I suppose," I said.

Nick looked annoyed or concerned, I never could read his face, and said, "Well god knows, you can't make him do anything he doesn't want to do, Mag. How long has he been talking crazy?"

"Maybe a week, but it didn't get really weird until the last day or so," I said. "He never sleeps more than an hour at a time, and he hardly eats. He's so messed up with pain and the drugs, he just groans and tries to move and hopes to get comfortable. But he can't."

Nick looked at the floor. "I've never seen him cry before."

I squeezed his arm and said, "This is bad stuff, Nick. The surgeon in Billings told me this spinal nerve malfunction makes pain that feels like fire. Fire, all the time, in his back and down his legs, and it never lets up. He's worn out and overwhelmed. His tears just reflect that. It's just been too intense, and he's been crying every day."

He paced a little and asked, "Are they going to keep him overnight?"

"I sure hope so," I said.

He looked at the time on his phone and said, "I gotta eat, do you want anything?"

"No, but maybe get something for Rock that he'd like."

Nick walked away saying, "I'll be back in a half."

I went to the cubical/room where Rockey was and the doctor was still there, but turned to me and said to Rock, "I need to talk to your wife for a minute; she'll be right back."

Rockey shouted, "She's not my wife, she's working with Nick to steal my stuff. Don't believe anything she says."

The doctor and I walked a little way down the hall, and he said, "Wow. I didn't find any reason to think your husband has had a stroke. He didn't know what day or what year it was, but on some things, he seems quite clear. He knows where he lives and who you guys are. He was very, very dehydrated. Has he been drinking any fluids?" I teared up and said I had lost track of his water consumption and asked if this was my fault. He shook his head and said, "No, no. You've kept really good records of everything going on with him. Don't make it your fault. It might be just a perfect storm. I am concerned about his kidney function, and we'll keep the IV in place and be able to measure his output. There's nothing in his records about these recent events. Where did he get that diagnosis?"

"In Billings from Dr. G. Do you want his number?"

He said he could get it, but he also said, "What do you want us to do?"

I repeated my thoughts about the oxycodone and Valium combination somehow becoming toxic. I said, "I think we should try a different drug." The doctor asked why Valium was prescribed and I described the spasms in his legs and sometimes his arms and told him, "The Valium worked better on the spasms than Flexeril, so they changed that a month or so ago."

"What do you think we could use instead and why?"

I told him about the test they did on Rockey a month ago, where they dosed him with morphine to see if he would be able to tolerate it when they installed the pump. He asked how that went. "He tolerated the morphine well and it did work much better on his pain; he seemed much less dopey in that twenty-four-hour period. Can he be switched from Oxy to morphine without suffering withdrawal symptoms?"

The doctor said, "I would think so, but I'll check with the pharmacy. Let me make some phone calls and I'll see you here in a while." I asked if he planned to admit Rock to the hospital and he said, "Oh yeah. We need to keep an eye on his kidneys and his urine output. He'll have to be admitted."

I secretly wanted to hug him just out of my sense of relief, but I just nodded and went back to Rockey. This normally soft-spoken, polite man had turned into a loudmouth, cursing guy with disdain for everything and everyone. I wasn't enjoying his transformation as he railed loudly about someone's odd shoes and the goddamn TV. He was pointing his hospital call remote at the monitor he was hooked up to and couldn't figure out why he couldn't find MSNBC.

Luckily, Nick returned with a bag of burgers and fries and was able to distract him from his current problems. Even though he hardly ate, I was grateful for any reprieve, however short-lived.

By the time the doctor returned, it was late afternoon and he told Rockey they needed to keep him overnight because his kidneys weren't functioning properly. The new crude version of my husband made some awful remark that shocked even me about the catheter, his penis and working kidneys and the doctor just chuckled and said, "Nope, the catheter stays in." Nick said, "I'll stay with dad tonight if you want to go home." He said he'd run home, then he and his wife Megan would be back by 6:00 p.m. or so. I said I would stay until he returned. Hospital time is different than the outside world and by the time they got Rock transferred to what would be his room, it was after 6:00 p.m. and Nick was texting trying to find us. I was so spent I just kissed Rock on the forehead, thanked Nick and Megan and headed out to my truck. I shut the truck door, had a big wailing cryfest, tuned off my phone and headed home, fell into bed with my clothes on and slept hard for a couple hours.

Prostitutes in the Basement

I woke up at midnight, intentionally avoided looking at my phone and snooped around for something to eat. I found some eggs and cheese, scrambled them, made some toast and fresh coffee. After a quick shower and a change into some soft clothes, an undershirt, and baggy shorts, I filled a travel mug, called up the dogs and walked down the half mile driveway. The night air was just right, cooled off from the heat of an August day, and it felt cool and clean on my freshly scrubbed skin. The moon was waxing but cast plenty of light to walk by. I stopped at the fence that runs close to the house and whistled softly while the dogs did dog things near-by. I could hear the horses coming before I could see them, the soft thuds of their hooves on the grass stubble, then as they got closer, I heard them breathing, then finally their low rumble of hello. I set my coffee down, bent and crawled through the high tensile fence and waited to be surrounded. I broke a cardinal rule by stepping into the horses' pasture with flip-flops on, but I knew they would be careful about my space.

With Lenny gone, the order for giving me affection had changed. Lenny was low in the hierarchy of the small herd, except when it came to loving on me. He claimed me as his own and made sure that he was front man when it came to hugs, kisses, and chest scratches. Bo had now claimed that spot and the others moved in at a respectable distance. There were seven heads to scratch, seven necks to bury my face in and smell their smell. I was rewarded by being welcomed and having my freshly washed hair smelled and tousled with soft, giant noses. Full up on horse love and their healing juju, I crossed back through the fence and continued down the driveway.

The dogs fell in, one in front and one behind, just happy as hell to not be in a truck in the hospital parking lot. We walked, kind of sauntered, with no real hurry in our steps. It felt amazing and I was vaguely successful at keeping the current medical crisis out of mind for one mile. But as I approached the house, seeing the lights on, I took a deep breath to face my future.

My phone had six missed calls, four from Rockey and two from a hospital number. Only the hospital left a message, asking me to call the nurses' station. It had been three hours since they left that voicemail, so I wisely decided to ignore it, thinking that if there had been something big, they would have kept calling. I was no longer a novice at fielding hospital calls in the middle of the night. I knew I wouldn't be sleeping anymore, so I grabbed a blanket and sat on the front porch all curled up and cozy. I tried to find that quiet spot in my head again but worrying had gotten ahold of me once more. I couldn't figure out what had gone so wrong in Rockey's head. He didn't show any signs of a stroke or other "brainstorms" as I often called them. I understood that the pain was outrageous, but I couldn't make the connection between pain and his crazy ideas. That left only the drugs as the culprit for his altered state, and the admitting doctor hadn't given me much support on that idea. I hoped they could come up with some answers for his increasingly erratic behavior, but I wasn't confident.

At 6:00 a.m. I dialed the nurses' station, wanting to catch the night people before they went off shift. The lead nurse for the overnight came on and proceeded to tell me what had happened. Rockey continued to be very agitated throughout the evening, becoming more vocal as evening turned to night. They continued to treat his pain with oxycodone and Valium, and there were no orders for morphine. He was very upset about the catheter and tried several times to remove it himself, but Nick had interceded.

However, Nick had apparently brought some liquor with him in his overnight bag and when Rockey continued his ranting, Nick, with quite a buzz on, began yelling at the nurses to do something for his dad. Nick was an intimidating guy when in motion. Just a mite shorter than his dad, at 6'2" and 250 pounds, with a rough loud voice and very big feet that propelled him in a rolling, charging gait, and none of the subtlety of his dad. The yelling Nick went down the hall to the nurses' station making such a ruckus, he woke up other patients. Meanwhile, his father was using a walker to escape to the parking lot to find his truck. A couple of nurses and a burly security guy corralled the senior Goertz boy and got him turned around back to his room, then politely escorted the younger Goertz boy out of the hospital and locked the door behind him. The security guy then took up a post in the hallway down from Rockey's room to help divert any of his mad dashes before he got far. My reaction was first to feel horrified at the escapades, followed by selfish gratitude that I missed the show. The hospital would not welcome Nick back, so I was now responsible to either stay the night with Rockey or hire someone to stay in his room as long as he was there. The hospital would not be responsible for his safety and would not allow him to stay without someone in his room at all times. Looking back, this was just a taste of what would be a challenging day.

I arrived back to Rockey's room right after the 7:00 a.m. shift change. It always took the new nurses a while to get around to all the patients they'd cover in a day. Rockey greeted me with a snarl and said, "Where the fuck were you all night?" I sighed and told him I'd gone home to check the horses, get a shower and a little sleep. "So, the horses are more important than me, huh?" I reminded him that "Nick and Megan stayed, and you are being cared for. Why are you so upset?"

"Well while you were off doing whatever you were doing, things didn't go so well in this hellhole."

I'd seen Rockey through some tough times as his body seemed to rebel at so many turns. He'd been confused, in pain, scared, hopeless, fearless and everything in between, but I hadn't seen this guy sitting before me now. This guy had a mean, squinty look, and his words were accusatory and martyrish all at once. "For one thing, everybody here is obsessed with my pissing. What the fuck is that about?" he said. I am an accomplished swearer and curse often and fluently. Rockey had never been much for cussing, and I was shocked he jumped right into using all the biggest swear words so often.

I tried to patiently explain, "Your kidneys are in trouble, Rock. They have to monitor everything in and out, so they can tell if the function is improving."

"I know how to take care of my own peeing. I don't need to be supervised," he said with his mean eyes narrowed and a nasty look toward me.

With only some midnight scrambled eggs and a moonlight walk between now and all the recent yesterdays, my patience didn't last. I walked to the side of his bed and lifted the catheter bag and said, "Look at this, Rockey. Your urine is nearly brown because you are so dehydrated. You quit drinking water because it hurt too much to walk to the bathroom. If we don't get this fixed and soon, you're not going to live to get that pain pump. You can't live with broken kidneys, and you need fluid to fix your kidneys."

His face fell, and he said quietly, "My dad had kidney failure. He hated dialysis."

"I know, Rock. You don't need that yet, but you have to let them try to fix you."

His combative guy returned, and he said, "I still hate it that everybody asks about my pee."

I stared at him for what seemed a long time and I said, "You have to be healthy in thirteen days. That means no infections and working kidneys, or they will postpone the pain pump surgery. I'm sorry that it sucks, but it's all we've got. Maybe they will switch your pain meds today, so you won't be so mixed up and you'll get more pain relief."

A nurse walked in just then and said, "Good morning, Rockne. I'm Kate and I'll be your nurse today," as she walked close to him on the other side of the bed.

He said, "Hey Kate, have you met my wife, Margaret? She's fucked everyone in Gateway while I've been locked up here."

I smiled sweetly and said, "Hi Kate, have you been to Gateway lately? Pretty slim pickins. I would have at least driven all the way to Bozeman if I was looking for that much fun." Dear Kate rolled smoothly with the punches and lifted the catheter bag and I walked out as I heard Rockey start swearing about everybody checking his pee. "I'll be right back," I said.

I walked fast to the parking lot and did my fresh air gulping routine as I made a quick spin around the lot. I returned to his room where Kate was still checking Rockey, and he was still being an ass as I sat quietly in a chair. At least he was just being generally bitter now, not overtly nasty. He did bring up the new favorite story that I was trying to sell his farm and steal his truck and on and on.

After Kate left and we ordered him some breakfast, I tried to find something on TV that might distract him. Rockey angrily launched into a story about the armed guard that was watching him last night. He told me, "The guard had a Billy club and a gun, and he swung the club at me."

I asked, "Where were you when he swung the club at you?"

"I was just walking to the door. I'm not a prisoner, right?"

"No, you're not a prisoner, but they can't let you go walking around outside at night when you're a patient. How did you walk that far anyway?"

He said, "I took a wheelchair and then found a walker in the doorway. I was almost outside when they caught me."

"What were you going to do outside?"

"Get the hell out of here, but somebody stole my truck."

"Rockey, nobody stole your truck. It's at home in the garage. And by the way, I don't think that guard has a gun or a club. He's here to keep you safe, not hurt you."

"What do you think, I'm stupid? I know you've got me locked up in here so you and Nick can sell the farm. Why can't I get some pain meds?"

"Let me go check," I said and swiftly left the room.

This was how the day went. And the next and the next. I "slept" in his room on a kind of lounge chair, and he never slept. He yelled and stormed and tried to leave, setting off a bed alarm that made everyone come running. He called me names and told all the nurses horrible things about me. By the third day, I was too exhausted to think, and I smelled like some old socks. I told the nurses I was going home to shower and change, and I would come back in a few hours. I asked them to make arrangements for someone to stay with Rockey and I would pay for it and that I would meet the overnight person when I returned.

I had just walked into the kitchen when Rockey called, screaming into the phone, "Where are you? You've been gone for hours!"

"I've been gone for a half hour, and I'll be back as soon as I shower, change and check the horses."

He started to talk about being locked up against his will and the horses being more important and I turned my phone off and got into the shower.

He was wild when I returned, frantically thinking I had left him. For the first time in a few days, I could see the fear back in his eyes. He really believed he was in some sort of prison, and although the morphine switch seemed to help with his pain, he remained firmly entrenched in this altered state. There was a doctor with him, and she told me they were baffled by his state. Kidney function was improving, but the fact that he was so agitated, so angry and so combative, didn't make any sense. I asked once more about the possibility of drug toxicity and got a blank stare from the doctor. No words. Just a blank stare. She was a petite woman and had been one of Rock's doctors in the mule-wreck hospitalization. Her lips were too big, like a fish, and she did the blank stare then too.

Abruptly, she said, "I want to do a lumbar puncture on Rockey."

I opened my eyes wide and said, "Why?"

She went on to say, "Well we just don't know what's causing this and maybe a lumbar puncture could tell us something."

"Like what?" I asked.

"Maybe he has meningitis," she replied.

I stepped a little closer and said, "He had a lumbar puncture two weeks ago in the Billings hospital. Where would he have gotten meningitis between then and now? In our home?"

She stammered and said, "Well we just don't know what's wrong with him."

I felt myself standing straighter and lowering my deep voice and said, "So you want to poke a needle into his spinal column because you don't know? He is scheduled for surgery to install a pain pump in less than two weeks. If he has even a hint of infection anywhere in his body, they will cancel that surgery. You are most certainly not going to stick a needle into his spine." She took a breath as if she was going to continue the discussion and I held up my hand and said, "Wait just a minute, please." I hurried out into the hall and asked a nurse to come with me right away. I got the nurse to face me and told her, "You are a witness. I am telling this doctor that under no circumstance is anyone in this hospital to administer a lumbar puncture or any other invasive procedure on my husband. Do you both understand?" I stood in front of Rockey's bed with arms out as if guarding him. They both nodded and the doctor walked out with the nurse following.

Rockey piped up then and said, "Why didn't they just ask me? I'd have said no way. You ever have one of those, Mag? They hurt like a sonofabitch."

The night watch person showed up a couple of hours later and I said goodnight and started to leave. Rockey started screaming, "Don't leave, Mag. They'll kill me for sure this time. Come back! Come back!" I was close to the nurses' station when I turned to look back toward his room and Kate, his day nurse, approached. She gently said, "Just go, Maggie. Go. He'll be all right. I'm working a double." Sobbing, I ran for the doors and home.

As I drove up the driveway, I slowed down by my little two-horse trailer. I thought I could load up Bo, throw the dogs in the truck and be in Idaho before anybody knew I was gone. I could find some more cash in the house, steal a license plate in West Yellowstone and maybe get all the way to Oregon. I was warming to the idea, but I knew I couldn't pull it off. Then what? I could never come back to the valley I loved because I'd always be the woman who left that sad, broken, nice man. I parked and dragged my tired ass into the house, warmed up a cup of coffee, rolled a fat joint and sat out in the last rays of the setting sun, wishing I was anywhere but here.

There wasn't much peace to be had. I had taken Rock's cell phone, but there was a landline in his room and the night watcher showed him how to dial 9 to get an outside line. By 9:00 p.m. he had called me four times. I called the nurses' station and asked them to secretly disable his phone somehow because if I didn't get some rest, I was going explode.

My phone didn't ring until about 2:30 a.m. I answered, and Rockey was whispering in the phone. "Margaret, you have to come back here right away. There's big trouble."

"What's going on?" I said in a sleepy voice.

Rock replied urgently, "You have to come right away and bring the sheriff."

I snorted and said, "Why?"

He got his very firm voice on and whispered harshly, "This is serious, Margaret! Listen to me. There's a Russian prostitution ring operating out of the basement here. That security guy is in on it. If you get the sheriff to come, he can bust the whole thing."

I perked up and asked, whispering too, "How do you know for sure?"

He said, "They asked me."

"They asked you what?"

"They asked me if I wanted a blow job," he answered.

"Well, what did you say?"

"Margaret! I said no, of course."

I answered, "Big mistake, big guy ... Just kidding!"

He was aghast but reiterated the seriousness, and I promised to call the sheriff. Instead, I called the nurses' station and told them I was shutting down my phone for the night and wished them good luck. I cried for what seemed like hours until I fell hard asleep.

Can't Stay Here

*A*s I rounded the corner at the nurses' station that morning, I was greeted by a cheery woman who introduced herself as something-something from Palliative Care. She asked if she could have a minute of my time before I went to see Rockey. We walked a little way and sat down in a cluttered office. After some pleasantries, she moved on to euphemisms regarding Rockey and his care.

Shrugging off my legendary tact, I said, "Please get to the point. So far, I haven't heard anything regarding Rockey or his condition or his care and I don't really understand what you're gunning for here."

She blushed a little and continued, "We can't continue to keep Rockey here. He is too combative and disruptive to the other patients, and we don't have the staff to deal with him. The doctors have no idea why his mind has become so altered and they also believe he may never come out of this state. I want to suggest two nursing homes in town that will accept him and who will take your insurance."

For once, I was too stunned to have a snappy response, but I could feel tingling in my arms and hear the roar of blood pumping in my ears. "How could they keep him safe in a nursing home?" I asked stupidly. "Can he go to one of the nice, new ones?"

She fiddled around with some papers and handed me a crappy flyer for the two places our insurance would cover. "The new ones are thirty thousand dollars a month for the care he would need and no, your insurance won't do that. These are the two you would be eligible for, and I encourage you to visit both today. I'd also like to invite you to the Parkinson's support group that meets on Tuesdays in the Aspen Point Day room." Another flyer slid across the desk, and I didn't pick it up.

I stood up and said, "I'm going to see Rockey now. I will think about what you've told me, and I'll be in touch. When does the hospital plan to kick him out?"

She blushed again and said, "He will be released tomorrow."

I could hardly breathe as I bumbled my way out of her office and back toward the nurses' station. I stopped there and asked, "Who has Rockey today?" They told me, and I went looking for the tall, beautiful, and most capable young woman named Julia. I found her and waited in the hallway while she finished up with another patient. I told her I needed to be gone for a while today and asked would she be able to handle Rock without me for a few hours.

Smiling kindly, she said, "I have a light load today and I promised I'd come by and tell him the story of my sheep hunt up Dudley Creek."

I softened and wiped a tear away and said, "Oh, you're the archery hunter. He told me he met you. We used to live up Dudley Creek, you know."

She said, "I heard, and I bet he has some stories too. He said you two had some wild adventures up there."

I laughed and said, "That we did, it was a one-in-a-million place to call home for a while. If you can get him telling those stories, he should be calm while I'm away. We had some big wild times up there where nobody but us traveled. We wouldn't see another human for days. It was awesome." A tear leaked down my cheek.

"Go take care of business, girl, I got this today," she said as she walked briskly down the hall.

I stopped into Rock's room where everything was the same. He looked at me with narrow eyes and started in about the pee watching and where had I been and why had I left that weird silent girl in his room all night. I started to cry and said, "How about not today, Rock? How about today you try being nice to me? I'm doing the best I can for you."

He sat up straight and yelled, "What the fuck do you have to be crying about? I'm the one being held against my will. You can come and go anytime."

I too straightened up and said, "You're right. I have things to do today, but I'll be back later. Julia is stopping in to tell you about her sheep hunt up Dudley. See ya." And I walked out, listening to his rants fade as I made for the door.

I was given the addresses for two facilities. I found the first one, an ugly, old brick building maybe from the forties, in a residential area not far from downtown.

There was no portico or covering on the entry, just an unlocked double door that led into an open area. Far ahead of me, residents were scattered about in wheelchairs or sitting by small tables playing games or doing crafts. In my near vision, an enormous man smiled through the glass door at me. He had twinkly blue eyes and a long snow-white beard that contained parts of maybe every meal he'd had for a few days. His chair was oversized, and he spilled from it everywhere. He must have been over 6'5" if he stood up. After the sweet smile and the twinkly eyes, the whole experience turned bad. I pushed the door open and was struck first by his shout of "HELLO!" immediately followed by the smell of urine so strong it made my eyes water and air so hot I couldn't stand it.

I abruptly turned and left before the door even had a chance to close.

Sobbing hard now, I drove fast for a little-used trail south of town called Indian Ridge. It was steep and shady, with not much for views, but had the prettiest little creek that ran through it. I hurried up the trail with the dogs happily sniffing their way next to me, and I stumbled down the hard hill, my tears making it difficult to see the trail. I pushed through the brush on a faint game trail, splashed across the creek and found a spot that I called the Big Flat. A completely flat rock about four feet in diameter that always held a little of the sun's heat in this cool, shady haven. I had found it a few years ago while picking huckleberries and I liked to think no one else used it because it was far off the main trail and kind of spooky in the brush. I took a big pull off my water bottle and yanked off my shoes and socks, stepping carefully onto the wet rocks to submerge my feet in the creek. I stood with tears streaming down my face until my feet hurt from the cold and climbed up and stretched out on my rock. Both dogs came up, snuffled my face, licked my tears away and went back to doing dog things. I laid there staring up at a patch of blue sky, peeking through the canopy for a long time, letting my tears run back from my eyes into my hair.

There was no way I could put Rockey in a place like that. I hadn't even bothered to go inside the other choice because I knew it wasn't an answer. I was so undone by my inability to figure out what to do. I maybe didn't always have the right answers, but I had rarely been so stumped by life that I couldn't even figure out which direction to go. I had proven myself able to handle Rock's physical disabilities, but I was pretty sure I wasn't built to handle crazy. For me, his current state was a horror show. I hated the yelling so much. The nasty stuff he said didn't bother me as much as it could have, but the yelling made me want to run.

Something broke in me that day. It was the day I said goodbye to any feelings of Rockey as *my person*. I was now his keeper and that came with a coolness, an efficiency unrelated to love but drenched in obligation and the need to do the right thing. I thought longingly one more time of racing down the road to parts unknown, dragging my little two-horse trailer with two dogs in my truck and a pocket full of cash. I shook my head at my silly little dream, knowing this was the day I would make the choice to stay and care for him until the end. This was the beginning of my season as a full-time caregiver, and the seeds of angry woman began to grow. That day Rockey quit being my person and started to be my charge. I did not welcome it and could not embrace these changes.

My feet had dried long ago, and I put my socks and shoes back on. I didn't know what time it was. A phone was of no use in these canyons, so I never brought it. The sun had moved past its high point, so I guessed it was early afternoon. I had found a decision on the Big Flat rock, and it sucked, but it was my decision. The dogs were finally worn out as we trudged up the big hill and back to the truck. I kept them with me as I headed to the hospital knowing I wouldn't stay very long.

I parked in the shade of a pitifully small tree, turned on some music and put the AC on high and left my sweet pals while I went in to tell the doctor what we were going to do about Rockey. I stopped at the nurses' station and asked them to find the all-too-cheery palliative care lady and the fish-lipped doctor and have them come to Rockey's room. Rock was a little less angry when I returned and retold a few of Julia's stories from Dudley Creek. I was relieved the yelling man was taking a break. Just about the time he started to wind up about being held against his will, fish lips and cheery lady stepped into the room. I didn't waste any time with pleasantries.

"I visited one of the facilities that our insurance has agreed to pay for and I wouldn't put my cat in that place. You can keep Rockey for one more night and then release him to me tomorrow," I said.

Fish lips looked surprised and said, "But he's dangerous, you can't take him home."

I stepped closer and said, "You haven't left me many choices now, have you? You're refusing to keep him, so I'd say you don't get a vote in where he goes once you throw him out. I've hired the watcher person to stay for the night and I'm heading out soon. I have a lot of things to get ready in order to bring him home. I'll be taking him out of here at noon tomorrow, please have everything ready for his discharge. We'll need two weeks' worth of morphine and Valium."

I walked over to the bed and leaned down and cupped Rock's face in my hands. I asked him how his pain was. "A little better today," he said. I kissed him on the forehead and told him "You're coming home tomorrow. No more yelling and don't make any trouble for the nurses tonight. I need to get the house ready for you and I've got some things to do so I'm going home now." He started to wind up with more crazy talk and I stood straight and said, "Tomorrow, Rock. You'll be home tomorrow and then you've got ten days until the pain pump surgery. No more crazy stuff or I'll make you live in the shop." I kissed his head again and said, "See you in the morning."

Deliverance

$\int$ wasn't willing to leave Rockey in the truck while I ran into the pharmacy, so there was time for him to become impatient waiting in his hospital room as I tried to get the prescriptions filled. It turned out that my regular pharmacy in the grocery store could not fill the prescription for morphine, so there was some wasted driving around and finally opening an account at the hospital pharmacy. I wondered more than once that day how the hospital could be so out of touch as to not be aware that only one pharmacy in town could dispense it and why that piece of information wasn't shared.

I was always amazed at the haphazard way someone gets discharged from a hospital. Even when the discharge is planned, it seems that everyone on the care team drops the ball simultaneously and are unable to make it happen anywhere close to the time they told the patient or the family. By the time I had the drugs and went to retrieve Rockey, he was dressed and sitting on the edge of his bed looking mad as a hatter. One of the many things he lost the summer he lost his mind was any realistic sense of time. Minutes were hours and hours were forever. From my point of view, the hospital had plenty of time to gather their discharge papers and orders, so when I sat with Rockey in his room for a few minutes and no one appeared to check us out, I went in the hall closet, got a wheelchair, and took control of his discharge myself.

The morphine had helped with the pain, but it was still ever present, and he moved stiffly to get in my truck. Getting off the oxycodone had not helped restore his mind and he was still fractious and unreasonable. He demanded that I drive around the hospital parking lot to look for his truck. He was sure that Nick and I had stashed it there when we attempted to steal it from him. I was apprehensive about taking him home, but at the same time I thought getting him away from the noise, the lights, the constant voices of the hospital, might help to soften the edges of his craziness. The doctors and nurses spoke often to me about Rockey being a patient with symptoms of extreme hospital psychosis, a psychological and often physical response to extended hospital stays. Although this time he was taken to the hospital for his rapid mental alteration, and the actual stay may have exacerbated his mental and cognitive decline.

He adopted a lecturing tone on the ride home, angrily declaring that I had locked him up against his will. At one point, he pounded the dashboard with both hands as he shouted at me. I was on a little country road with no one behind me and I slammed on the brakes and very quietly said, "If you do that again, you can find your own ride home. I won't sit two feet away from you when you're acting this angry." He stared at me with his angry eyes, and I held his gaze and he finally said, "Okay, sorry. Just take me home please and I won't do it again."

Once again, I got him set up in his big recliner in the living room, turned on the TV, got him some water and gave him his phone. I thought he would want to call his kids or Tim when he got settled, but he didn't. The pain was returning, and I started a new section in the growing drug diary, making all the accompanying notes on his status as we started this new path with morphine and a different muscle relaxer for the spasms. The morphine was liquid and dispensed orally in a tiny amount with an equally tiny syringe. He opened his mouth like a baby bird, and I squirted the relief under his tongue. The good thing about morphine was that it acted quickly. The bad thing was that it didn't last very long, so the drug schedule changed dramatically, and I felt some pressure to make sure I wasn't going to overdose him. I had put all the new drugs in a green ceramic pitcher and hidden them in a pretty display cupboard we had. About three hours after we got home, Rockey decided he wanted to be in charge of his own drug regimen. It was his tone of voice and way of speaking to me now that always set me on edge, no matter the content of his words.

He barked at me in his bossy voice, "I should have all the drugs right here by my chair. Why are you putting me through this, having to ask every time I need them?"

"I'm not sure you're in the best shape to be monitoring your drug times, Rock. What did we have for lunch?" I asked.

"What does lunch have to do with it?" he yelled.

"I don't think you can remember lunch or what we had or when we had it. I don't think you can manage the timing of these drugs. I am trying to keep you safe."

He started pounding the arms of the chair as his anger whipped up and said, "I don't need you to keep me safe. I can be in charge of my own goddamn drugs."

I stood in front of him and thought about the uselessness of arguing with someone whose brain had left the building. I was tired physically. I was tired of being screamed at. I was tired of being the grownup. I turned and walked to the cabinet and got out all the drugs and the tiny syringes. I picked up the notebook that contained pages of writing, logging all the drugs for the past seven weeks, and I carried the whole mess over to him. I had never shown him the drug log and even in his confusion, I could see the surprise in his face at the amounts of drugs he had been taking. I handed him the notebook and put all the bottles in his lap.

I said, "Here you go. This is the history of what you've been taking since June, and these are the new drugs. They have a completely different schedule. It's all written down on the last page." I grabbed my phone, walked back and snapped a photo of him with all the stuff in his lap.

He asked, "Why did you take a picture?"

I said, "When I have to call Nick and tell him that you've overdosed because you insisted on being in charge, I want to be able to show him this picture of you taking control of your drug schedule. I have to go do chores." I left and walked slowly to the barn, hoping chores took an extra-long time tonight.

It looked to me as if some horses needed brushing, so I got my wish, hanging out with my quiet, lovable giants for a while. Somehow, the decision that I had made while lying on the Big Flat rock had brought about a change in my way of coping with taking care of this broken man. I felt less guilt being away for a little longer. I felt less pressure to endure his rants and get whatever he wanted in that exact minute. He was no longer in an acute medical situation. His pain would remain unchanged until he got the pain pump installed, and I was doing all I could to mitigate that pain while we waited. It appeared that the loss of mental acuity was not going to change. I had enormous concerns about living with this new crazy person. Only because his physical ability had become so diminished, I wasn't afraid of him that way. But the constant anger, paranoia and yelling was draining me, and I had no interest in engaging with him to try to talk sense into him, firm in my stand that you just can't argue with crazy people or drunks. He would demand answers to his loony questions in his angry voice, and I would answer with, "Oh, sure," or, "I don't know," just to pacify him.

While I felt less emotionally whipped, my new position of keeper was an odd, empty place. I had loved Rockey so completely for so long, this felt like I had just dropped the rope that tethered us together. There was a bit of relief in letting go of the emotional attachment but with that relief came the knowledge that things in my house had forever changed. He looked like the guy who stole my heart, held me close, made me laugh, took me on fine adventures. He looked exactly like the guy I had upended my life for, the same guy who I was always so happy to see at the end of every day. He bore a striking resemblance to a man I had made love with, in our bed, in our kitchen, in the woods, in tents, on the river and in a whole bunch of model homes. But that man didn't live here anymore. This was a guy in a Rockey lookalike suit who screamed, thought I was a criminal, believed I wished him harm and generally found new ways to verbally assault me.

That confusion in what I thought I saw and what was really there was the truest heartbreak I ever experienced. I had to remind myself that it wasn't fair to be angry with him because he had no control over what he had become. In a normal relationship, we are allowed to be angry when our partner treats us badly or unfairly. With a little skill and a little luck, we are able to navigate these stumbles and come through them with a better understanding of each other. There was nothing normal between us anymore. He was a very tall and huge angry child, and I was in charge of keeping him fed, clean and controlling his pain. I was his advocate and his decision-maker for all things in the spaghetti-shaped medical world. That I can name the week, the date that this all changed for me, that I let go of being in love with him, that I let go of any dreams of future adventures, sweet nights in the wilderness or flying down a mountain in a cloud of powder snow, sitting in the moonlight in the hot tub counting shooting stars, riding horses to hunt for horns in the spring and being transported by the beauty of these hills, that I can say the day this all went away and I became his keeper and began a period of mourning for a live person, will remain my greatest heartache. I had packed my broken heart away to become a sure and assertive advocate and give this man the best care I could.

When I got back in the house, I entered through the laundry room, so I didn't have to walk by Rockey, and started making us something to eat. After a few minutes, he called my name and I walked over to stand in front of his chair so I could look him in the eyes. He pointed to the side table where he had neatly lined up the drug bottles and the syringes on top of the drug log notebook. "I think you better be in charge of this. I don't even know what day it is." I nodded and said, "Okay. If you need more of any of it, just tell me. I won't keep it from you just to be mean, you know." It was his turn to nod, and for just a second, I saw a gentle look in his angry eyes. I gathered up the drug supplies, put them into the pitcher and back into the pretty cabinet.

There wasn't anyone around who I felt could help with watching Rock while I ran to town. He was too aggressive and mean for me to ask any of my friends. He had shown me that he had the capacity to talk his male friends into doing stupid things that left me picking up the pieces, so I wouldn't ask them. I did try to hire some help from the local home healthcare companies. I arranged for two different agencies to send a person to our house so we could interview them to help with Rock's round-the-clock care. The first one was scheduled to come at 11:00 a.m. Rockey wanted to be awake, so he declined his scheduled morphine at 10:30 a.m. When she still hadn't arrived by noon, he threw in the towel and asked for his dose. The woman finally came up the driveway at 12:30 p.m. and I was sitting on the front steps.

She introduced herself, and I said, "What happened? Our appointment was for 11:00 a.m."

She smiled and said, "Oh, I went to lunch first."

I stood and said "Thanks for making the drive. I can see you are not the person we need for Rockey's care. I'll be calling your boss to let her know why." I went back into the house and found Rock fast asleep in his chair.

The second potential helper made an equally poor first impression when she showed up on time, but in what was obviously last night's clothes. She smelled like she'd slept on the floor of the bar, and I think was sporting a little bit of vomit on the front of her satin jacket. My opening line was, "So, tell me what it is you like about doing home health care."

We were still standing out on the sidewalk in front of our house and she kind of looked at the ground for a minute before answering, "Well, it's just a temporary gig for me. I'm trying to get a job at the nursing home, but I have a suspension on my employment record."

I smiled and said, "Good luck to you, but I don't think we'll be needing any help after all." Again, I turned and went back into the house, figuring I was going to be handling this without help.

The days ticked slowly by as we waited for surgery day. Rockey was still held captive by the immense and unyielding pain. There were no nights when we both slept undisturbed. His once sharp mind was a jumble of darkness, self-absorption, and a just plain shitty attitude. I gave him whatever he needed: his meds, good food, fresh clothes, and we did the awful hard dance into the shower every other day. I would ache for hours after helping him in and out of the shower and back into clothes. Every so often, I would forget where we were in this life and would try to start a conversation with this guy in the Rockey lookalike suit. It nearly always led to Rock going off on some paranoid accusation, and I would silently walk out of the room, shaking my head at myself for not knowing better.

The day finally came, and I drove the 168 miles from my door to St Vincent's Hospital in Billings and two much-diminished people entered the hospital to register Rock. I pushed him in a wheelchair into the elevator, and the door opened near the check-in desk. Dr E's assistant was just about to get in the elevator and stopped and turned and exclaimed, "Oh Maggie, I'm sorry, I didn't even recognize you two. Rockey, how are you? You have the pain pump surgery today? I believe Dr. E will be in the surgery suite with you." I nodded and gave Rock the space to answer her, and he replied nastily, "It's about damn time. I'm nearly dead." Standing behind him, he couldn't see my face and I gave her an eyebrow lift and a tiny head shake. She put her hand on Rockey's arm and smiled sweetly and sincerely saying, "I know it's been a terrible ordeal, but they're going to get you feeling so much better."

I helped Rockey register, as he couldn't remember his birthday or his social security number, or where he lived. The check-in lady said someone would be out to get him in a little while, and I rolled his chair out of the busier area of the waiting room. I excused myself and found a restroom. I locked the door and splashed water on my face, trying to breathe deeply to find some calm at the start of what promised to be a long hard day. The woman I saw looking back at me in the mirror as I dried my face and opened my eyes shocked me. No wonder the assistant didn't recognize me. I had dark circles under my eyes and my cheeks were sunken. My already weathered face had become even more lined, and it looked as if I had aged ten years. And my hair was a bad mess in need of a cut right now. Splashing more water on it didn't help my ruined face, and the deep breaths weren't cutting it either, so I returned to the oh-so-familiar waiting room, hoping they called him soon, thus ending my watch for a while.

They called his name, and I wheeled him back to the surgical prep area, where a nurse took over the driving as soon as we crossed the threshold. He was allowed to take his regular doses of morphine that morning because the intrathecal pump would not be effective for twenty-four hours. Rock was nervous and rightly so. Dr. S, the Pain Clinic guy, stopped in as well as Dr G, the neurosurgeon. A Medtronic rep was also part of the entourage. I started to step back so they could get closer to Rockey in the small room when Rock reached for my hand, which was remarkable only in that he had not exhibited any tenderness toward me for weeks. I took it as fear and neediness but was glad to offer this poor guy whatever comfort I could. They explained the procedure yet again. The pump itself was an oval-shaped thing, about four inches long and three inches tall, that went under the skin just below his rib cage and a little to the left.

From the pump, they ran a wire and a catheter under the skin, just to the left of his spine, where a small battery would sit. The wire connected the pump to the battery, and the catheter snaked past the battery and would run up next to his spinal cord where the opening would end just above the inflamed nerve bunch. When it was activated, the pump pushed an amount 1/300th as much as an effective oral dose of morphine through the catheter so it bathed the inflamed arachnoid in a continuous morphine drip. By applying the morphine directly to pain receptors, the brain was fooled into thinking there was no pain, and even though it could never remove all his pain, his life would be more bearable. He could manage the remaining discomfort, mostly with ibuprofen. Rock became a little fixated on this part as the doctors were speaking and asked in his bossy voice, "Well how much pain are we talking about?" They explained again that it was hard for them to paint a picture of such a subjective thing as pain. I left the room in my mind for a bit, not needing to listen to another impossible conversation, until I thought it had gone on long enough. I squeezed Rockey's hand and said, "Rock, it's okay. It's the only thing we have left to try; you can't keep living like this. Any relief will make it worthwhile, and we'll just deal with the rest of it." He pursed his lips and shook his head as if he thought he deserved a more definite answer. The doctors seemed relieved, and the Medtronic lady stepped up and told Rockey that she oversaw the mechanics and would be turning off the neurotransmitters in his brain so they could get the scans they needed to work on his spine.

Rockey's eyes grew wide, and he said, "Oh, don't turn them off. I don't want to know."

"Oh, Mr. Goertz, you won't know," she said. "I won't turn them off until you're under anesthesia."

Rock's eyes filled with tears, and he repeated softly, "I just don't want to know."

Again, I stepped back in and gently stroked his shoulder and said, "You'll never know, Rock. They'll make sure. She knows what she's doing."

With the neurotransmitters turned off, his Parkinson's tremor would become visible, and he would be faced with seeing the progression of devastation that had continued even though it had been masked from him for five years. That's what he didn't want to know. It took all I had not to shudder at the thought as I tried to reassure him. Finally convinced enough to let them go, Rock returned to his apprehensive waiting until a kind nurse showed up with some light pre-op sedation. This had always been my cue to leave, and I leaned in for an awkward hug and kissed him on the forehead. "I'll see you in a little while." I made sure the nurse, the anesthetist and doctors all had my cell phone number before I walked out. It would be at least three hours before he was in a room, so I drove through a coffee shop and got a triple latte and a dried-up slice of lemon poppyseed cake and headed up 27th to the Rimrocks.

I got lucky and found an area with no people and carefully set up my little spot on a ledge. I put the cake on top of the little bag it came in and spread out a couple napkins. I found a smooth spot to set my coffee and got comfortable in a lotus position. I hadn't planned this funny ritual, but it felt right to have a little moment of kindness to myself. I looked out over Billings and the treetops and tried to feel the freedom in knowing that for at least three hours, nobody needed me, and there was nowhere I had to be. Ultimately, I decided three hours wasn't nearly enough to get silly about, and I was happy to eat cake and enjoy the high-test coffee in peace.

Rockey was a real mess when they finally got him into recovery. He was very confused and having significant pain. It took a couple of tries for me to figure out that it was both pain at the surgical sites and the continuing pain in his back. I remembered from his DBS surgeries that the wires—and now the catheter—being pushed through muscle was a terribly painful experience. The pump morphine wouldn't be effective until tomorrow at best, so he was truly miserable. I went to find the nurse and wasn't surprised to find out there were no orders for any pain meds for him. There wasn't much I could do beyond pester the nurse to pester the doctor who would be stopping by "soon." Even writing about being with Rockey while he had intractable pain makes everything in my body grow tense. There would never be a distance so great between us that I wouldn't be physically affected witnessing his pain with no comfort to offer. I never grew accustomed to that helpless feeling, and it slayed me every time.

Dr. G finally did stop by. He issued an order for something other than morphine for pain, concerned about the clash of oral drugs and the new pump-delivered drugs. Rockey was released, and because it was late in the day, I got us a room at the old Clocktower Inn and ordered some bad Chinese food. We didn't eat much. Rockey was not only in pain and still living on some other planet, but he was also in that weird, agitated state that seemed to be caused by anesthesia. It was the tail end of a very long road, and I was out of everything. I gave him what I had for his pain, but it didn't help. I called Dr. G. When he called me back, I was circling the parking lot smoking cigarettes I bought off a drunk guy sitting in the alley.

"What can I do? What am I supposed to do? Could they help him if I took him to the ER?" I asked.

Dr. G quietly replied, "There isn't any more we can give him today. I'm sorry, Maggie, I am surprised by his level of pain. But there isn't anything we can do; he's just going to have to ride it out."

I can't say I was surprised to hear that Rockey was maxed out on drugs. I did feel a new kind of deflation as I said, "Okay, doc. We'll get through this night, and I'll take him home tomorrow. Thanks for calling back. Good night."

He responded, "I'll see you in a couple weeks. It will get better."

I went back to the room, and Rock was immediately loud and demanding about his pain. I grabbed a pillow and a blanket and put them on the very small, upholstered chair. I stood by the bed and looked at my husband and said, "I spoke to your doctor. There is nothing more you can take today. The pump will kick in tomorrow, and then we can start giving you something to relieve the surgical pain. But tonight? There is nothing. No more. I need you to stop talking and if you can't sleep, I need you to be quiet. I absolutely have to sleep to be able to drive us home tomorrow. I'm going to sleep in the chair, so you can move around in bed to try to be comfortable. I'm not mad. I am exhausted and there is nothing I can do to help you tonight." He nodded and turned onto his side. I curled up in the chair and later moved to the floor. I didn't hear any more sounds from Rock. Whatever we had couldn't be called good sleep, but at least there were no sounds of pain.

I woke up wearing my clothes from yesterday, brushed my teeth with a hotel toothbrush and washed my face and called it good. I helped Rock to the bathroom once more and back to the bed. I asked him to wait for a minute and I ran down to Stella's and got us coffee and two big fat cinnamon rolls. With a lot of sugar and a little caffeine in our bellies, I got us loaded up and headed for Gateway.

On the way home, I called Nick and said, "We'll be home soon. I need you to come and stay with your dad for the rest of today and overnight. I'll make sure you have something for dinner. I'm leaving at noon and I'm going to the cabin. You can take care of him for twenty-four hours. Okay?"

Surprisingly, Nick said, "Sure. I'll be there."

About an hour into the two-hour-and-forty-five-minute drive I dug around in my counsel and found a bottle of Advil. I shook three and handed them to Rock pointing to the water bottle in his side door pocket. He was all done being quiet about his discomfort, and I kept chewing up the miles as he bounced from one wrong thing to the next.

I know Rockey was as relieved as I to be home. The sad dogs were so happy that their people had returned. I got Rock settled into the bed, turned on the TV and went off to fix some food for lunch and for them to have for dinner. In between food tasks, I gathered up supplies for my overnight. I didn't need much. Rock was finally sleeping soundly in the bed.

Nick rolled in just after 11:30 a.m. and Rockey was just about to
have a sandwich, so I made one for Nick too. While they were eating, I grabbed a fast shower and put on some clean comfy clothes,
threw my bag in my truck, loaded up the dogs, fixed myself a cup
of coffee for the road and turned to tell the boys goodbye. I gave
Nick an easy rundown, "No drugs, only Advil, and he needs to
rest. Drink water and rest. I'll be back by noon tomorrow," and off
I went.

The tiny cabin was cool in its deep green woods. No running water, one bare lightbulb, a wood stove, and an old electric range. No
telephone or cell service. I started a pot of coffee and gathered up
some wood. The dogs were happy snuffling around in the woods
and dipping into the creek. I set my tiny speaker on a stump,
turned on some music from my phone and built a little campfire.
The coffee was ready, and I put some cheese, crackers, and olives on
a little plate, rolled a joint and took it all out to the little fire. I sank
deep into a camp chair, put my boots up on a log and just sat there
enjoying my treats. I got the dogs to sit on the crooked bench and
tossed them cheese bites and tried to get a picture.

There was no epiphany. No special rays of sunshine beaming
down on me. I was an aging beauty whose face had been worn out
from riding through hell. I was edgy and felt kind of mean-spir-
ited. Soft music, Tom Waits, a toke now and then, a little coffee warmed up from the pot by the fire and the low water of the
creek whispering through the trees. My sweet dogs checking in
from their adventures making sure I was still where they left me.
I breathed it all in and a tiny bit of tension and angst left me with
every exhale. I went in the cabin to find those awful marshmallow
cookies from the little market in Big Sky. Throw a little sugar in
this deal and you've got a real party, I laughed to myself. More
wood, more fire, more weed, and more coffee.

Then a real sad song came on by Amos Lee about a burden and
that was it, the tears finally came. It wasn't the huge sobs I'd been
expecting, just a sad unending flow of tears that lasted until the

moon was high. When the crying finally stopped, I doused the fire, called the dogs and we went inside. I crawled into my bed heaped with down and fleece blankets and slept for twelve hours. Uninterrupted for twelve hours.

Nothing Worth Remembering
Fall 2014

In the aftermath of the summer of 2014, the pain, the drugs, the crazy shit started to feel less like sharp things in our lives. The pain pump started to do its job and Rockey became more comfortable. The surgical incisions started healing and caused less distress after a few days. There was a silence in our house that I had missed. During that silence I thought about the past several months and the challenge of how we got here.

The episode of pain which began in May of 2014 ramped up to full-throated screaming pain in June. He had started taking opioids then and was finally diagnosed in July. By the time Rock suffered his psychotic break in August, he had been heavily medicated for nearly eight weeks. The surgery to install the pain pump finally came in late August, and was effective at minimizing his pain within a few days. His recovery from this whole episode was long and slow. By this point, he had regained normal kidney function, and his appetite returned although it was not as robust as it had been. Rock weighed about 205 pounds before the summer of 2014, and that might have been a bit more than he liked. By summer's end he was down to 185 pounds, which was his normal fighting strength.

In his torso, he carried three Medtronic devices implanted under his skin, which improved his life. Two batteries for the neurotransmitters in his brain—one just below his right-side rib cage and one just above his left collarbone—were hooked to the transmitters by wires that snaked under the skin to his brain. Now he sported the pain pump which was also just below the skin and under his rib cage on the left side. At 205 pounds, these devices were barely visible when he had his shirt off and the wires were completely undetectable. Now, at this lower weight, they had become a prominent part of his physical landscape. Neither of us thought much of it because the batteries and pump were just part of keeping him comfortable, and vanity seemed superficial when considering quality of life.

Rockey's post-surgery demeanor was radically different than the guy I lived with for the previous four months. His voice and speech returned to his hushed tones, and he seemed almost apologetic for a while, with a wide-eyed look most of the time. He was easily tired and mildly confused by too many ideas in a sentence. Gone was the rage and that high level of anxiety produced by the inescapable pain. He was subdued. Archery season for elk hunting had opened, and by the third week of September, he was ready to go to his hunting shack to watch for elk. I was delighted that his interest was rekindled as it was his favorite season, and I loved the optimism it took to be a hunter. This year, as in recent past years, I was surprised and grateful that when Rockey set up a target to practice shooting with his bow, he was still a bull's eye shot nearly every time. I knew if that skill returned each year, he would have something to be happy about and feel masterful.

Autumn remained a good time to be Rockey. Even in his diminished state, he was diligent about putting in his hunting time and was rewarded with taking a 5 x 5 bull elk. That measurement refers to an elk's rack of antlers. It means this bull had a medium to large rack with five points or tines on each side. In a hunter's world, it was a respectable size. He didn't have the strength to field dress it, but called our neighbors Ron and Suzy, who showed up to help him with the task. As always, if there were more than two people, I was content to be in the background and see the joy on his face as they joked and laughed through the process, and that he had those moments of accomplishment to enjoy. He thanked our friends and sent them off with whatever quarter of elk they most desired.

The fall of this year was peppered with doctor visits for Rock. He did not feel that he could drive safely, so every two weeks I drove him the 332 miles roundtrip to Billings to see one of his many doctors. Dr. S, the Pain Clinic guy, wanted to monitor his acceptance of the pain pump and the continuous morphine now streaming into his bundle of angry spinal nerves. The doctor asked many questions regarding the level and type of pain Rockey was still experiencing. He explained that there were thousands of combinations of drugs that could be administered through the pump, and although the relief would never be 100%, they could find the recipe that gave Rock the best results. About a month after the initial implant, the doctor suggested changing the mix from pure morphine to a combination of fentanyl and morphine to better treat the still significant pain he had in his legs. Rockey did feel less pain in his legs, but by day four with fentanyl, he started to feel bad. He was nearly panicked when he told me, "Something is wrong. I feel so weird, kind of dizzy and weightless and really messed up. I gotta get this drug out of my pump." I said, "Well, let's call the office and tell them what's going on. You can't be the first person to have a bad reaction to a drug." I dialed and ended up leaving a message to call back, which didn't happen.

By the next day, Rock was approaching hysteria because of the "weird feeling" that he was not able to specify. Once again, I dialed the Pain Clinic office and handed the phone to Rock. He spoke to a nurse and explained his troubles and she said, "We can get you in and remove the fentanyl in two weeks and go back to straight morphine." I heard his voice rise a bit and he said, "I can't wait two weeks, I'll be dead by then." They went back and forth, and she explained the reason for the two-week wait was for ordering the drugs and that they don't keep a supply on hand. Rock pleaded and I thought he laid on the drama a little heavy, but he wasn't at all threatening, just more like a martyr. By the end of the negotiation, he was able to get in a week sooner.

He really did feel horrible and slept most of the time until I was able to take him in. We were taken back to a tiny exam room and met by a very stern-faced Dr. S. He looked straight at Rock with angry eyes and said, "If you ever talk to anyone here in that tone of voice again, we will end our relationship with you. You do not make our rules and you cannot bend our rules." The admonishment went on, and I left the room in my mind again, as I've done so often before. They changed Rockey's drugs, and he was feeling better within forty-eight hours. He was so scared by the doctor's lecture, he never again reported any problems with his pump, and there were troubles along the way. I couldn't disagree with his decision to keep his mouth shut because of the threat of discontinuing service. However, I thought it was poor form to scare a patient with chronic pain into silence for the sake of compliance. I never accompanied him to see this doctor again, as I didn't trust myself to comply with silence and acceptance orders. I would drive him there, but I never went in the building.

He also needed to see the surgeon several times during the last quarter of the year. The site of the pain pump had healed well; however, because of Rockey's twisted rib cage from the mule wreck so many years ago, there were problems. When he installed the pump, the doctor used the same measuring formula he did for all patients receiving a pump, and with Rock's odd ribcage shape, that position was not working. When he bent over, his lower rib would rub against the pump. Dr Goodman was kind of surprised and said, "Well I'll be damned!" when Rock stood up and demonstrated. We all agreed to wait for Rock to continue to recover but scheduled another surgery to move the pump down by a few inches.

As Rockey slowly regained some strength and stamina, his mind was not bouncing back as well as we had hoped. He lacked clarity of thought. He might have an idea of something he wanted to do, like a project in his shop. He couldn't collect his thoughts to explain that project to me. He might name it but would search for terminology that should have been familiar to him to describe his plan. This became frustrating for him because he said it made him "feel stupid. I just can't find the words." It made him reluctant to speak, and it seemed to rob him of confidence to plan things. He felt he could never grab up all the pieces of thoughts he needed. It's difficult to describe, but the best way he explained it was, "If you think of a plan like a paragraph, it's like my paragraph has things blacked out in it. I don't know if they are important things or not." I thought that was a succinct description for a guy struggling with clarity, but it always left him feeling that he had forgotten something important.

Rockey was softer in the aftermath of the terrible summer. His endless drive to be busy, to be in motion, to be productive, had waned dramatically. It wasn't just that he was tired. A flame had been extinguished. He cried easily and often and was always embarrassed by his tears. I tried to tell him he had suffered some terrible losses and raw emotions had to be a part of his recovery. I told him that women could cry and not feel judged, but we accepted our own wailing as a cleansing thing. I tried many ways to ease his embarrassment over his tears, but in the end, I don't think my words could hold candle to our cultural expectation that men don't cry. More is the pity for that myth.

One night in late October, we were in the hot tub watching for falling stars and he said softly, "I don't remember anything."

I asked, "Anything about what?"

He waited a moment and went on: "The last thing I remember was the day they tried to give me a cortisone shot in Bozeman. I remember screaming and asking them to stop. I remember you being mad. And I know the pain never went away after that. Did I start taking Oxy then? When was that?"

I was stunned by all this, and I had to take a minute to remember what month it was. "I think it was late May or maybe early June and yes, that is when the Oxy started."

He stared at the sky for a while and quietly said, "Falling star. I have three."

I turned my eyes to sky because it was an on-going competition and said, "There's one. I have two."

"What month is it now?" he asked me.

"It's October, Rock."

I heard him take a deep breath and could see him looking at me in the moonlight, and he tentatively asked, "Can you tell me what happened? Would you explain to me how it all went so wrong? I just don't remember anything except feeling like fire. Like I was on fire. What happened to me and why can't I remember?"

My heart felt like it was going to explode and all I could hear was the blood pounding in my ears. I was glad for the night so he couldn't see the sadness in my eyes or the tears that now fell. I couldn't imagine where to even start. I said, "Do you know about the arachnoiditis?"

He said, "No. What is that?"

I explained in the best shorthand way I could the definition of the disease, the chronic inflammation of the nerves in his spinal cord, and the pain it caused him and that the only fix was the pain pump. I asked him if he could summon any memories at all.

He thought for a bit and said, "I remember a guard. Was I in jail?" I told him the story of him believing that he was being held against his will and that they were going to kill him. "How do you know they weren't?" he asked. I sighed and tried to change the subject, but he brought it back with, "I do remember the prostitutes in the basement. What about that?"

I chuckled and said, "That wasn't real, Rock. You were hallucinating."

"Nope," he argued. "That was real. I know it was. You were never there and that's why you don't know."

"Careful," I said. "I was there every day, Rockey, and most of the nights. If you want to have this conversation, don't begin by telling me what I didn't do for you. Because I do remember."

We both took a moment and took a few breaths. He started again, "Okay. I don't remember you being there. I remember you leaving and screaming for you, but you never came back."

I was silent for what seemed like a long time but probably only a minute or less. I realized that he was just so mixed up … so unaware of the magnitude of what the summer had been like. It made me sad for a selfish reason: we would never have a conversation about the terrible, awful, horrible thing we endured together. We did endure it and came out the other side, but the story we each told ourselves shared no common victory. I decided right then, I would never tell him the whole of what had happened. I didn't believe he possessed the emotional tools to process that information. I could not have told the whole story without telling him the ways he wounded me. His denial of those wounds would have been like being back in the middle of it.

So instead, I told him, "Rockey, there is nothing about the summer of 2014 that is worth remembering. You had intractable pain caused by a rare disease called arachnoiditis. It started in the spring, and we went everywhere to try to find out what was causing it. Everywhere we went, they were unable to figure it out, but they gave you painkillers, mostly Oxy. The pain got worse and finally Dr. G got a scan and saw that the nerves in your spine were all messed up. Then you got the pain pump and started to feel better. It was a horrible experience, and you just have to believe me when I tell you that it's better if you don't remember. Nothing good happened all summer."

He was just looking at me with a sad look and I saw his eyes start to sparkle with tears. He finally reached across the water, took my hand and said, "I'm sorry, Mag. For whatever happened, I'm so sorry."

I slid across the hot tub and into his lap, wrapped my arms around his head and rested my head against his and said, "Thanks,

Rock, but you had no control over any of the things that happened. Neither of us owes the other an apology. It was just a cascade of very bad things, and we did what we always do, the best we could." We sat like that, crying softly in each other's arms, him trying to remember, and me hoping to forget.

Trying to Find Me
2015

As the year 2014 finally came to an end, Rockey had resumed driving. He had the surgery to move the pump in early February and in the scheme of things, it wasn't a very hard recovery. He had some pain at the incision for a few days, but felt great relief from the new position, so he deemed it a success. He sporadically lifted some weights and worked at improving his mobility by walking to the shop, about a quarter mile. That short walk usually caused his legs to feel stiff and sore so he never could get in the habit of doing it regularly. Hence, he never saw the improvement he hoped for. He used his walker around the house for a while and then I saw it tucked in a corner of the garage as he started using a cane. He preferred the cane as it didn't shout DISABLED as loudly as the walker, and he became proficient with it as an aid. It continued to be uncomfortable for him to sit in a hard-backed chair, so we ate our dinner in the big recliners in front of the TV and forever abandoned placemats and table settings.

The changes to our life were small if I look at them one at a time, but over time, in order to compensate for his deficits, there were many of them. Somewhere in the past, he had become the dishwasher unloader, for which I was unreasonably grateful because I hated the task. Now the bending and twisting motions were too painful, and the job came back to me. Small change. It was nearly impossible for him to put on his socks so I helped him whenever I saw him struggling with it, but he wouldn't ask me to help. Small change. He didn't trust his ability to get in or out of the hot tub or the shower without assistance. Small change. I removed end tables and bookshelves from the living and dining room area, so he had a straight runway from the bedroom to the kitchen with nothing to maneuver around. Small change.

I can easily admit that none of these were life-altering changes, but to me, as they added up and Rockey's need for my assistance increased, I began to feel squished. I imagine that caregivers across the world feel the same fading of themselves as the demands on their time and energy increase and the reciprocity fades. In the moment, I couldn't name the exact feelings or the exact cause, but I found myself becoming an angry and impatient person. By spring, I could hardly stand my own thoughts plagued by anger and a pissy attitude. I looked for a business card I had kept from an encounter years before. I had been in a Pilates equipment class. It was mostly the same women, three days a week for a couple of years. I was, of course, the class clown as we sweated and struggled with good form and proper posture and engaging those core muscles at just the right time. We all worked in front of mirrors, and I was the oldest by some margin. I would shout out as we neared the ever-changing last repetitions "Oh my god, I can't believe my boobs look this bad in active wear!" or, "Why didn't you guys tell me my ass had disappeared?" or, "Seriously, can anybody really make their foot go that way?" and they would all crack up and lose their concentration. In this class, there was a petite but strong woman who came in late every session. Once as we were leaving, I stuck out my hand and introduced myself. She smiled broadly and said, "I know who you are. You're the whole reason I never miss this class." We both laughed and I asked her what she did. She told me she was Amy, a counselor specializing in clients with life-altering diseases like M.S. and Parkinson's, and I stopped listening and interrupted her by saying, "Perfect! What serendipity!" She was always in a rush to return to her office, so I asked for her card and gave a brief explanation of Rockey's condition and said, "I might need to call you someday." Not long after that, I quit the class.

Someday had arrived, so I found her card and I left her a message that started with, "I'm not sure if you'll remember me ... blah, blah, blah, but I'm in trouble and I could use your help." When I answered her return call, she said hello and laughed a full but gentle laugh and said, "Of course I remember you. Class has been boring since you left." I made an appointment, and I was looking forward to this new path with a new light to shine on my life. It took a few sessions to lay out enough background for her to have a clear picture of Rockey, his increasing dependence, his decreasing abilities and me with all my issues. On her intake form, the last question was "What do you hope to gain from these sessions?" I answered, "I want to find a way in this caregiver role to handle it with grace and dignity. I want to be able to look at this part of my life and know that I did it well, that I offered the care and advocacy that Rockey deserves. I want to try to remember what it was about him that I ever loved. I want to quit being so angry." And off we went on one of the best journeys I've been on.

To say Rockey had become self-absorbed would be a gross understatement. Through my growing resentment, I began to wonder if he had always been so, and did I just never notice? Had he been more clever at hiding it when he possessed all his marbles? How much had I contributed to putting me far down on a priority list by waiting on him, by seeing to his needs and by coordinating all his medical stuff? In the aftermath of the terrible summer, I was lost. I had hoped for a bigger recovery. I had probably convinced myself that more of the man I had once loved would return when the pain and the drugs diminished. I might have believed I could reclaim some of myself, the Mag who had some friends, some fun, some laughs. I grabbed on to the fact that he had never put my name on the deed to the farm and swirled it around in my head, feeding the growing knot of pissed-off person I had become.

My self-loathing grew as I began to see myself as little more than a servant who lived in a nice house, with little control over my life. My time was taken with caregiving. I couldn't be gone for more than a few hours at a time because he couldn't be trusted to not get in trouble with anything from the kitchen stove to trying to fix the baler. His judgement was so poor and his denial so great, he was like a ten-year-old boy. He was emotionally inept at anything regarding our relationship. I chose my words with care to avoid riling up his paranoia and never bothered to initiate any constructive conversation about where we found ourselves. He seemed to feel he was owed everything I had to give and was free from all rules of reciprocity. I was too tired, too frayed, and too disappointed to do any more than just get through the days. I woke up every single day with the same thought. I would open my eyes and say, "Oh fuck. Another day." It was a dark, dark time for me, and I shudder to think what I might have become had I not found Amy.

I saw her twice a week for many months. I never cried in our sessions, but recited facts and hurts with the same flat reporter voice. She commented once about my objectivity. I took it as a compliment. Amy shook her head and said, "No, Maggie. It's not good. It may have been good when you acted as Rockey's advocate. It may have served you as you navigated the perils of the medical system. But here? Now? In this room, you don't have to be objective. You can unlock all those emotions you've put away. You were excellent at guarding Rockey. You did what you had to do to protect yourself by shutting all your feelings away. But if you hope to walk out of here someday different from the person who first walked through my door, we're going to have to let those things come out."

I stared at her and stared some more and finally said, "I don't remember how. I only feel angry or flat. I don't even know who I used to be."

She looked at me with her big, bright intelligent eyes and said,

"I knew her, and I can help you find her again. She's in there. She never left. Are you ready to move forward?"

A single tear ran down my face and I said, "Yes. Let's find her and bring her home. I think I liked her better than this chick."

My sister Kathy was planning a road trip from Wisconsin to visit that spring. This is the letter I wrote but never sent a few weeks before she was to arrive:

Dear Kath,

I hope this finds you well and enjoying spring.

I'm writing to tell you some things I need you to know, but couldn't trust myself to speak them without falling apart. You need to know that you are coming to a house of great sadness. Rock has suffered so many losses and continues to lose ground almost daily. His life with three progressive, incurable diseases is a slow, sad theft of his dignity, his strength ... his sense of self. While he has days where he works in the shop on stuff and he goes fishing now and then—he rarely smiles, speaks infrequently, and has moments of overwhelming fear and grief and tears over his inevitable future of further losses.

I am just trying not to be lost. I do nearly everything for him and feel compelled to be available much of the time. There are days when I am away for a few hours, but that has become more of a rarity. I am incredibly sad. I have a good therapist and she is trying to help me hang on to me.

I have withdrawn intentionally from most of my friends here. I just can't find enough in me to participate. I do not wish to be the sad girl that everyone wishes hadn't shown up.

My shrink told me it was important to tell you what you are

*in for. She thought I would call you, but as I considered the con-
versation, I could only weep. This is not anything like you may
remember. It's a house filled with despair and naps and an occasional comfortable moment. This isn't even one of the crisis moments. Our life is mostly about pain and disability.*

*So, there you have it. You are always welcome in my home.
I think it will be a very sad trip. Or ... maybe he will find his
magic by then.*

I love you, Kath. I miss simpler days.

I didn't send it because I thought this was just the beginning
of how life was going to be. It wasn't going to be better by fall or
by next year. Kath came and stayed. We stuck close to home. She
had always had a decent relationship with Rockey, one of the few
people in my life that he trusted enough to speak to and hang out
with now that he was someone else. I had worried ahead of her
visit that having another person in the house would add stress,
but I should have known better. Kathy glided in, made herself at
home and we shared some laughs, some stories and good food.
The familiarity of her love and companionship was soothing and I
missed her company when she left.

Rockey had planned a fishing trip to Fort Peck Lake in eastern
Montana with his brother Tim and his old partner and good
friend Tim Klosner. Those two would drive from Minnesota with
Klosner's big fifth wheel camper and Rock would drive the seven
hours from here with a camper and the boat. I had doubts about
his driving so far with such a complicated towing set-up but kept
my worries to myself. I helped him pack and did his supply shopping for him. I was surreptitiously keeping an eye on him as he
made his preparations and he seemed to be remembering all the
tiny details he needed to be ready. I had to hand it to him; I didn't
think he would or could pull this trip off, and I was hopeful that it

would all work out. Anything he was able to master independently would contribute to his confidence and overall well-being, thus making this house an easier place to live. The *Tims* would be there to help set up the camper and launch the boat. I was positive the boat launching was not something he could handle on his own. There would be too many times getting in and out of the truck, getting in the boat while it was still on the trailer, bumpers out, tying off … this list of small tasks is long, and he was not up to it physically. The best part was that the *Tims* were two of his longest and best friends. Klosner called me before they arrived and asked what he needed to know to be able to help Rock. Tim Klosner was and is a fine human. He and Rockey ran their business, hunted, fished, golfed, laughed, drank, told stories, made trouble and just hung around since they were teenagers. In my eyes, they were lucky men to have had such an enduring friendship. When Rock was diagnosed with Parkinson's, all the retirement plans got moved up. We moved to Montana, and Tim and his wife built a house on a lovely lake in Northern Minnesota where Tim got to fish all he wanted. We would see them occasionally, and Tim came out to hunt elk with Rockey, but their time together was scarce and limited. I always noticed in those years that Tim was like a balm for Rockey's soul. It occurred to me that, beginning with their shared youth, together they were a force and maybe some of that shared strength or history of accomplishment or just plain trust seemed to give Rock a steadying hand when they spent time together now. Quite simply put, Rock was better when Tim was around.

Alone Together
2015

Rockey drove off with his too long load of camper and boat and I crossed my fingers that he was up to the drive. There isn't much cell coverage by Fort Peck, but he called when he was about an hour from the campground. Rock said he had pulled over and napped at a rest area and was feeling good. He had gotten texts from the *Tims* and knew they would be there before him. That is the news I was hoping for so I could quit picturing him stumbling or falling trying to set up all by himself. I was grateful for four days of nobody asking for anything. I planned to stay up late, play music loud, sleep late and have olives and cheese for dinner if I wanted.

My long-time riding pal Karen was packing up their home not far from me because they were moving to St George, Utah. We shared an odd friendship, and I was damn sad she was leaving. Truthfully, I was more than sad. I was bereft. She was smart, older than I, a prickly, never-hugging kind of woman with a wicked sense of humor. We shared the same lefty political views and a lot of good jokes about growing up Lutheran. She was organized and a concrete-sequential thinker and I was not that. I always wondered how she could manage loving me, random, chaotic, creative person that I am. But she did. I taught her to say *fuck* more often and showed her that pink and orange flowers do look fabulous together and she tried to teach me how to organize my spice cabinet and convince me to make better passwords on my computer. We rode horses hundreds of miles together over the past eight years and she listened to my trials with Rockey's care and still felt affection for him. We had planned our last ride together that week and we both showed up wearing better clothes than usual, so we'd look good in the photos. I cried and wanted a hug. She cried and complied the best she could with her stiff arms banging on my shoulders.

I was grateful for my solitude later that evening as I sat on the porch, thought about our last ride and reminisced about time and trails together. Karen had been a sturdy post in my support system, loooo as it was, and I knew I was unlikely to ever find another like her. I had compiled a big mess of photos of our many mountain adventures, laid them out with text telling the story of our friendship and had a book printed and bound for each of us. I drove to her house in the middle of the night, slipped through the locked gate to her place, and put it on the seat of her truck so she could find it when she was leaving. She called me crying from a rest stop in Idaho, bitching because she didn't get me anything, but with gratitude in her voice. It was a perfect Karen response. I miss her still.

Rock's fishing trip was a success. They only caught a few fish, but lots of big belly laughs for the fellas. Rockey didn't drink much anymore, and he said the *Tims* were sad about that, but he pointed out to them that he walked like he was drunk all the time, so they could just pretend. I thought it was funny. Tim Klosner made plans to come that fall for elk hunting from the shacks on our farm.

The summer was quiet. Rockey was uncommunicative and seemed to be in his own world much of the time. I couldn't guess whether he didn't tell me things from his life because his need for secrecy was growing, because he didn't remember, or because it was so taxing to form thoughts and put them into words. Whatever the reason, we spoke very little.

I continued seeing Amy at least weekly and occasionally twice a week. Rockey's recovery seemed to have stalled or have gone as far as it was going to go. There seemed to be huge blank spots in his knowledge base. Things that had been routine in terms of his motor skills were becoming more difficult.

Parkinson's patients experience a thing called "masking." The medical community thinks several things contribute to it. First, these patients are either without any or have a synthetic supply of dopamine. Dopamine, in addition to being a neurotransmitter, is an essential part of a human's ability to feel pleasure or have the drive to want pleasure. Masking is simply the absence of facial expressions. The lack of facial expression makes communication dicey, as often Rock's words were not given any help by his eyes or his mouth smiling or frowning. Just listening to his words, I was often unsure whether he was experiencing something bad or good, so when he came out one morning and said, "I can't run a toothbrush anymore. I can't do the brushing motion. Do you have more brushes for the electric one?" I said, "Sure I do," and hopped up to show him where I kept the spares and how to use it. He was so matter-of-fact with his declaration, I didn't respond with anything more than to find the brushes he was looking for. I made no acknowledgement about the loss of this motor skill. Later, he told me that my lack of reaction hurt his feelings, as if I didn't care. There was no good that could come out of my explaining that his flat affect led me to believe it wasn't a big deal to him. There would be many such miscommunications in our future.

Seeing Amy was beginning to help me with my feelings of rage and helplessness regarding my loss of identity. She tried to help me make plans to combat both. I talked often about my load of guilt for having my fantasy plans about running away. I discovered that running away fantasies were quite normal for caregivers, and that guilt was unnecessary junk to carry around. We talked about Rockey's self-absorption, and I spoke about my demotion to servant, instead of feeling like a partner. She helped me learn to adjust my expectations because first, it's normal for a person who is losing their physicality to become focused on their own losses and ways to either deal with those losses or find a way to circumvent them, and second, it was no longer personal, his disregard for me. Without dopamine and with having reduced serotonin levels, his brain simply didn't have the capacity for love or concern or humor or much of anything that didn't relate to him. So, while we occupied the same home, and I cared for his needs, I felt alone. Rockey had no interest in my day, my adventures, my struggles, my injuries. He mostly wondered what we were having for dinner and what was on TV. I acknowledge that I had always been comfortable being alone and had never felt lonely. This was different somehow. Living with someone who was half of what was to be a pair, and who had taken an emotional leave from that pairing, felt lonely. Living alone by choice sounded much less painful than being alone in a house with someone else. It created an edginess that I felt and could only quiet by going outside.

I began to fill up my time rather unconsciously with activity to divert my attention from the air of misery in our house. I had been hiking alone for years and it was great for me physically, mentally, and most of all, emotionally. Now I added some goals to the hikes. I planned to hike twenty-five miles a week and see what happened. It became a tonic for all the ragged edges in my person. My legs only took me to places where there were no people. I had no desire to share this time with anyone. I got to be in excellent shape and found more peace than I could have imagined thumping down some beautiful trail talking to the dogs. I marked my mileage on the calendar each time I went out, curious to see what else I might gain from it.

As summer turned to fall, Rockey found his focus for elk hunting and his aim with his bow could still shoot an arrow true. Devoted archery hunters are a bit of an uncommon breed, and there are less people who use a bow and arrow than there are gun hunters. He most often hunted alone in the shacks he had built on our farm, which happened to sit within an elk corridor. To bag an elk with a bow, an archery hunter has to be much closer to the elk than a gun hunter. Rock's shots were true up to sixty yards, but a good sportsman never wants to risk wounding an animal with a bad shot, so he most often waited for an opportunity to take a shot at less than fifty yards. The key word there is *waited*. I haven't known many hunters in my lifetime who hunted every day of a big game season besides Rockey Goertz. He went every afternoon during the seven-week archery elk season. This year, he was once again able to walk to his shacks, which were about six hundred yards from the house. It was a big physical win for him after the bedridden year of 2014, and it seemed to bring a sparkle back that had been missing for a long while. The walk wasn't easy. It took him a long time to get to the shack, and it was tiring for him, but the good outweighed the bad and he persisted.

When the gun season opened, Rockey decided to join his friend Bob and some others to hunt elk up the Gallatin Canyon past Big Sky in some national forest land. Bob had a little primitive Forest Service cabin very close to ours, and the old boys packed up food, beer, and horses with a plan to stay for a while. I helped Rock get his good horse Pancho all ready to go, making sure he had all the tack and supplies he might need for cold weather riding. After a couple of decades together, there wasn't much Rockey could surprise me with in terms of what I liked to call his Big Ideas. This one shocked me. He had only ridden one time, early in the spring that year. He asked if I would take him out for a ride in the hills that May, to see how it felt. I tacked up his horse for him, helped him into the saddle, and he rode with a rookie's death grip on the saddle horn. I rode behind to keep an eye on him. His balance was so poor, I was concerned he might slide off.

We rode up some steep terrain while Rockey looked for elk horn sheds, and I kept my eyes on my unsteady husband. We were only out for about an hour when I noticed his posture began to change.

I suggested we head home before he got too tired or uncomfortable. It looked to me as if he barely made it back to the barn as he slumped and fidgeted in the saddle. I was wildly relieved that he hadn't fallen off and I didn't have to try to get him home again from a wreck, a sad milestone for a guy who used to ride dozens of miles in a day, pulling a string of mules. So great had my anxiety been on this little outing, I promised myself that I would never take him out riding again without someone along for backup.

So, when he announced that he wanted to take his horse up into the forest and hunt from horseback, I was blown away. Snowy ground, steep canyons with shaded trails, bitter cold air and the promise of lots of getting on and off a horse sounded beyond his capabilities. True to my promise to myself to not let my fears for his safety get in his way, I did all I could to set him up for a successful trip. I knew that Bob and the other guys would watch out for him, and I was glad his safety wouldn't be my responsibility.

With no phone service in that part of the canyon, I didn't expect to hear from him for a few days. Like always, I took advantage of the fleeting solitude. Rock drove up the driveway four days later without the horse trailer. He had come back for a doctor's appointment in Bozeman and was smiling when he told me he was having so much fun, he intended to head right back to the cabin after the appointment. Again, I was stunned but happy to see him enjoying himself.

The weather turned colder, and Rock came home a few days later. They had not found any elk, but his subdued demeanor suggested something greater than that was on his mind. I unloaded Pancho, put the tack away and helped gather up the dirty clothes and hunting gear to bring to the house. Rock showered and laid down to rest.

During dinner that night he said quietly, "I fell off Pancho."

To my knowledge, the only fall off a horse that Rockey had ever experienced was the huge, bucking wreck from the mule a few

181

years prior. But with his poor balance and lack of confidence, I wasn't completely surprised. I said, "Tell me. Are you hurt?"

He shook his head slowly and said, "No, I'm okay. We were on that trail passed the abandoned camp, you know where it curves and gets steep?" I nodded. He continued, "I was leading, and we were riding down. When we started around that curve, it was shaded and super icy. Pancho was slipping toward the mountain side, and I just slid off and rolled down that steep bank to the creek."

Picturing the bank and the creek in my mind, I said, "Jeez! That's quite a tumble, Rock. How did you get back up and why didn't you get hurt?"

"I had on my big Carhartt suit, and the snow was pretty deep, so I didn't land hard. Bob and Clay had to crawl down the bank to help me back out and then it took both of them to get me back up on Pancho."

I was trying to minimize his humiliation and said, "It's almost impossible to swing a leg over the saddle in one of those big suits."

"Yes," he said, "it is. But the truth is, I didn't have the strength to pull myself up into the saddle, so they had to push my ass up to get me in it. It was awful."

There wasn't anything I could say that could fix this. I touched his shoulder and said, "I'm sorry that happened, Rock." I picked up his plate and his glass and took it all to the kitchen and started cleaning up. In my head were the thoughts about knowing this day would come when another thing he had loved to do would face a forced retirement. Through my counseling and through necessity, my efforts to maintain objectivity were working. Although I recognized another loss for Rockey, I no longer felt the emotional tug of grief for these inevitable losses. This was both a comfort to me to spare myself the sadness, and at the same time it felt as if I was cheating the process of loss somehow. I took that for what it was.

. . .

A couple weeks before Thanksgiving, Tim Klosner showed up, and he and Rockey busied themselves in their Boys' Hunting World. As I mentioned, Rockey was always happier and sharper when Tim was around. They hunted here on the farm, and Tim was fortunate to snag a big bull elk. It was below zero when I went out to take some photos of the smiling hunters with their frozen breath in every shot. I wonder if I had known that it would be Tim's last hunting trip or Rockey's last horse ride, would I have taken more time to soak up those feelings that sprinkled hunting season with other people's joy? Would knowing it was the last of a long line of hunting seasons have marked it somehow for me? As it was, I was happy to see two grown men who loved each other dearly spend time together as they had so many times before.

For a while after elk season was over, he was optimistic. There was a determination as he resumed his yoga /stretching classes. He began to do his old exercises for his back and strength building.

Almost instantly, it seemed to unravel. There was no remarkable incident. He started to tire more easily, needing more sleep. I don't know if he was aware, but his mind seemed to be muddled. There were more things forgotten, like discussions about money that went wrong, because he had no idea what our income really was. In early December, we had a conversation about our upcoming cruise to Alaska's Inside Passage. We talked about it being very expensive and perhaps too ambitious, as it included hikes and kayaking. We threw around ideas for an alternative trip—the Keys, Southern California, or Utah. In January, his credit card was credited with a portion of the down payment on the Alaska trip after I cancelled. Somewhat aghast, he had no recollection of the conversation. I began to see that he was deteriorating at a more accelerated pace. Even after the yoga, the supplements, the forced walking, and additional sleep. Despite the neurotransmitters, the pain pump, the prescriptions—both used and refused—he began to lose ground. His lurching gait turned to a shuffle almost overnight. His speech grew quieter and more difficult to understand.

As these things were happening, he must have been frantic. He spoke of wanting the doctors to turn off his pain pump because he thought the morphine was paralyzing his legs.

We were in the hot tub one night, and he said, "I want them to turn my pump off." I know he said more but I was not hearing him. My reaction to those words was visceral and immediate. I felt my stomach flip, saw stars and had ringing ears and a racing heart. Remembering the weeks before the pain pump and the agony he experienced threw me back to a place best left forgotten. I took a deep, slow breath to quiet my rising panic and selfish thoughts and asked what he was hoping for.

"I can hardly walk anymore. My balance is terrible. I feel like I'm going to fall ninety percent of the time. It has to be the morphine. I think they should turn it off. I think my back is better." I started to talk about Parkinson's and its progression. I reminded him that arachnoiditis never gets "better." Then I stopped. Realizing all the reasons why I couldn't be discouraging to him at that moment. I said, "Well, let's get some appointments with your doctors and see what they can tell us."

With the phone calls made and the appointments on the calendar, I hoped that someone we would be seeing would have the courage to tell him what I could not.

Journal Entry

2/3/16

1:26 a.m.

I am not sure.

I am not sure who I want to be in this. No, that's not it. I am not sure what I'm so afraid of. Am I afraid that he'll find a surgeon who will perform some surgery and that surgery will not help him and the recovery will take more than any operation can return to him? Or am I afraid that what I have thought for some time is true. That there is no return for Rockey. Soon he won't be walking. Then will he have a wheelchair or a scooter? Will he need help all the time? With everything? Will we need to have someone—a caregiver—live here? How will he handle this? More anger, depression?

Will he finally give up? Should we build a ramp off the front porch? Should we sell the farm and buy something more manageable?

Who do I want to be in this?

I want to be courageous and helpful. I want to be strong and empathic and thoughtful and kind. I want to find good answers and solutions for the trouble he will face. I want to be patient. I am sure of this.

I feel like I don't have enough left to be all those things. I want to be solitary and self-indulgent. I want to take road trips and hike in new places. I want to accept a spontaneous invitation to something. I want to lay on a beach and get sunburned and not care. I want to not feel stuck.

I know I'll wake up tomorrow and say the same thing I say every day: Oh fuck. And it won't matter that I don't have enough left.

Baby Love
2016

*A*s the new year began, we made no resolutions. Both Rockey and I still carried the scars of the past in our lingering exhaustion and ebbing hopelessness. There were plenty of doctors' appointments, and I usually drove Rock to Billings. Since he resumed driving, I had not ridden with him and didn't plan on it. The trip to Billings in winter was often over icy roads, with high winds and reduced visibility. As much as I had grown to hate the trip, I couldn't abide cutting him loose to drive himself. The Pain Clinic continued to check the volume of morphine, and Rockey was approaching the time when the batteries for his neurotransmitters would need to be replaced. Life was quiet and sad, each of us searching silently for something to embrace or look forward to.

Rockey was keenly anticipating the birth of his first grandchild. Nick and Megan were due to deliver a baby girl in January, and Rock dreamt of little girl outings and the impact he would have in her life. I held him back a little from visiting the day of Andi's birth, saying, "It's their first day with their new little person. Let's give them twenty-four hours to have her all to themselves." Megan needed an emergency C-section, and they were longing for a

186

bit of quiet to recover. When we did make the visit to the hospital, Rockey was overcome with joy.

He took that baby in his arms and sat on the little hospital couch with her and seemed to get lost in searching her tiny, perfect face. He smiled softly as he whispered to her. His eyes were brighter than I had seen them in years. He just stayed transfixed by Andi and looking at her every detail. It was a lovely moment to witness. One of the best photos I ever took was of him cradling this tiny being in his giant hands, looking down at her with pure love. The pregnancy had been a difficult one for the new parents, and they were looking forward to settling into their home with some baby routines. I was happy for everyone's elation but felt little connection to the joyful group. After years of them pushing me out of the tight family circle, I was content to stand on the edges, try to honor their joy and risk no more rejection.

I spent some months thinking about hope during this time. My conclusions were probably jaded by some standards. I came to believe that hope was indeed a necessary feeling to be able to push forward through challenging times, but I couldn't help viewing it as a double-edged sword. Rockey hoped to find a cure for all his ills. He hoped a doctor could magically perform a surgery that would restore the mobility he was losing almost daily. His hopes pictured mountain adventures like his old days and some powder-filled skiing excursions. He had no middle ground. My hopes for Rockey looked more like adaptation. I hoped he would lower his work benches in the shop so he could continue to do projects but from a sitting position. I hoped he would say yes when I sent him one more link to a motorized cart that could take him safely into the high country again. Our hopes for his future were so disparate, conversations about the future were limited and often punctuated with irritation toward the other's ideas. He would talk to me about looking for one more surgery that might restore whatever it was he believed was possible, and I would temper my reactions with neutral noises. When I sent him links to the newest inventions to enhance a disabled person's mobility, he would wordlessly delete all those links. He stubbornly and proudly refused to consider using anything that smelled like a wheelchair.

We went to the doctors' appointments he insisted on that were silly and a grand waste of time. Imaging showed his knees were fine, as were his hips. The only spinal surgery that might have helped was one not performed on a man of his age in generally poor health. I cornered the two neurology doctors on one visit, out of hearing range of Rockey, and said, "You guys have to tell him. It's your responsibility to tell him that no surgery will fix what's wrong. That he isn't going to find a miracle cure for what is stealing his life. It can't be up to me to tell him these things. I'll just be seen as a negative wife. As long as nobody ever says the words, he is going to keep shopping for surgeons to do something to 'make him walk again.' It has to come from you guys."

They nodded, and one of them said, "Maggie, you can't discount the importance of hope in his life."

I replied, "Hope is one thing. Being attached to unrealistic goals is a completely different thing. If no one is willing to tell him the truth, I promise you, he will arrange some dangerous procedure in this quest to be whole again."

They nodded some more and walked away. No one ever told Rockey the truth about his condition. His life became this weird seeking of some magic surgery that could save him, make his pain leave, and allow him to hike up a mountain again.

Baby Andi came every Wednesday for about four hours. We played little people games and were both delighted by her laughter. Rockey would hold her sweetly in his lap and read books to her. He was still able to be on the floor and they were cute and smiley together. As time went on, he began to resent or be jealous of the physical things I could do with her that would have her squealing with delight. I could carry her and toss her and take her down the driveway to visit the horses. When he began to be snarky about the attention I stole from him, once again I retreated to the *Keeper* position. I changed diapers, fixed tiny-person snacks, filled sippy cups and reduced my one-on-one time with Andi to almost nothing, so Rockey wouldn't feel threatened that this child might like me better. His needs were greater, and my joy was the sacrifice.. Her company brought him all the joy he had in his life, and I was grateful she was that gift to him.

The winter following 2015 was quiet, with no new surgeries or health issues. My mental health continued in a downward spiral, and by May of 2016, I felt desperate. I finally confessed to Amy that, "No, I am not doing all right. In fact, I cry every day. Sometimes I cry for hours. I can't find any hard reason and I can't find any way to come out of it." I admitted to feeling like I was drowning in sadness, washed over with my helplessness. We talked and we talked, and Amy finally suggested that she thought it was in my best interest to start taking some serious anti-depression drugs, instead of the low dose of anti-anxiety meds I was taking.

"Why? Nothing has changed," I argued.

Amy said, "You can't stop crying, Mag. That is new and it is not in your best interest to leave it unattended."

I started to cry again and said, "But why? What changed or why did it change?"

She told me that I had fought for Rockey like a warrior, putting all his needs ahead of my own during his months of psychotic break. "That was incredibly traumatic and now you're left with the grief. Your future is clearly not going to be what you ever hoped for. You can see nothing but the escalation of Rockey's care needs. You are grieving the future you will never have and the loss of your partner and your friend."

I disagreed with what I saw as the drama in those statements, but I reluctantly agreed to get a prescription. It flattened out the few highs and any happiness I might have found, but it was successful in pulling me back from drowning in hopelessness. Emotionally flat had become my goal. Yuck.

The future plans Amy mentioned were real. Rock and I had intended to spend our retirement years adventuring. We had talked about doing extended pack trips into our favorite wilderness places and were excited to explore new backcountry. One solid plan was a longer trip into the Bob Marshall Wilderness to camp near the iconic Chinese Wall. We had tried once before but were turned back before our destination by six-foot snowdrifts in July. Our plans included winter trips to a few more exotic spots for scuba diving. A six-week road trip to Alaska was among the most ambitious dreams. The list of fun was detailed and expansive and every one of them was never going to happen.

In August, Rockey decided to build Andi a toy chest. It was a simple wood project for him, and he was happy about his idea and excited to be in his shop building something again. I was working in the vegetable garden when I heard his truck honking and driving quickly up the driveway. As I ran to the truck, I saw he had his door open and his left hand in the air wrapped in a filthy shop towel.

"What happened?" I asked, seeing blood running down his arm.

He said, "I really fucked up this time," and I unwrapped the towel. His hand was laid wide open from the space between his little finger and ring finger, across his palm and all the way up his forearm about eight inches.

"Stay put and I'll get a fresh towel." I ran into the house, got the towel, locked the dogs up and ran back. The arm was dripping blood onto the ground as I gently rewrapped it. I helped him into my truck and slammed it in reverse out of the garage and started driving crazy fast down curvy backroads heading for the hospital. I asked him what happened.

"I was cutting the pieces for the toy chest and a piece of wood bucked. I stumbled forward and put my hand out to keep from falling. But I put it right into the saw."

"Did you have a guard on the saw?" I asked.

"Nope," he replied.

At this point I asked him how he was doing, and he seemed to be fading. I grabbed his arm, lifting it and reminded him to keep it up in the air. I called 911 and told them I was racing toward the hospital with a very bad saw injury and wanted to get the admittance information out of the way so they would take him right back for treatment. The 911 dispatcher asked if we needed an ambulance and I told her I thought we'd get there okay. I answered a few more questions about Rockey and then said, "Oh no, he's passed out. Can you have the ambulance meet me at 19th and Stucky? I'm three miles out." She said they would be there, and I stepped harder on the gas.

The ambulance and firetrucks were waiting, and I thumped my truck into the ditch next to them and jumped out. A firefighter grabbed me by the shoulders and said, "It's okay, ma'am, we've got him now."

I said loudly to him and the EMTs, "He has Hep C—be careful. His name is Rockey. Rockey Goertz, 12/12/52, and he has a thick file in the ER."

They laughed and gloved up, lifting Rock into the bus, and the one that had ahold of me had me sit down in the grass. He took my pulse and said, "Well, you're fine. I heard the recording of your 911 call. I'm guessing this isn't your first rodeo with bad accidents. You were amazingly calm and gave us every piece of information so clearly."

I snorted and smiled and said, "Yeah, we've done this all before, I guess."

He asked me to sit with him for a minute and said again, "They've got him now. They'll take good care of Rockey. You did great. Just sit here for a minute until you're sure you're okay to drive. I'll drive the rig in front of you with the lights on and we'll get there about the same time as they do."

It was a busy time of day for traffic across the MSU campus, so I was happy to tuck in behind the big red truck parting all the obstacles. We did indeed pull up to the hospital just as they were wheeling Rockey past the intake desk. I thanked the desk people for expediting him and helped them fill in the rest of the information. By the time I got back to Rockey, they had cleaned his wound, used a topical anesthesia, and lightly covered it with gauze. He had been given some pain meds and was sitting comfortably in a room, waiting for the on-call orthopedic doctor who specialized in hands. I don't recall whether it was through a text or a phone call, but we weren't there very long before my friend Lori showed up.

I had known Lori for at least a decade. She managed a wonderful tack store and western boutique with all kinds of great treasures a girl like me would love. She had helped Rockey shop for me on many occasions in his physically challenging years. Lori never spilled the beans to me that a gift from the store was coming my way but did tell me when I thanked her for helping Rock that she thought he was a lovely man. She was always so touched at the thoughtfulness he put into finding something for me. He would call her and ask her if she had time to help him, show up at the store and she would have a spot ready for him to sit down on. He always had something specific in mind and asked if I'd shown any interest in something. Lori liked that he never asked her to pick something but took time to look at things to find just what he had in mind. It was a kind of Team Shopping and I always benefited from their efforts.

Rockey had been a champion gift shopper in his mobile years. Contrary to some of his steamrolling tendencies, he loved Christmas and birthdays and put huge effort and thought into presents. In the years of his struggles, he had Lori wrap things at the store, but for twenty years before that he stalked the perfect gift, bought paper and cards, and loved making a big presentation of his finds. He had listened to me through the year and would find that one weird thing I'd talked about and would never have gotten for myself. Rock loved overbuying for everyone he loved. The best part of this Christmas extravaganza was that he wrapped every gift for every parent, sibling, and child we bought gifts for. We set everything up on our dining room table and I would box things and scribble a name on the box, and he would wrap—beautifully I might add—and attach the name tags. It was a helluva production in our big holiday days, and we both got pleasure from the giving.

Lori hung out with us while we waited, and she offered to do my evening chores if I was at the hospital too long. When the hand doctor came in, she quietly moved away from the bed and listened while Rockey and I talked to the doctor. He was handsome and cocky and a little over the top with his arrogance. Cocky Doc, as we started calling him immediately upon his exit, entered the room and introduced himself by saying he was "the best hand doctor in town and good-looking too," flashing a Hollywood smile. He was excited about the gore of Rockey's wound and asked if he could take some photos to share with other doctors. "They won't believe this," he said excitedly. I was already becoming annoyed with his approach but held my tongue. He set down his phone and picked up Rockey's arm, probing the wound gently, but with ungloved hands. Then he finally turned and scrolled on the computer screen, reading Rockey's information. He shrieked, actually shrieked, "OH MY GOD! You have Hep C! How could you not have told me? Oh my god! You could have infected me! I can't believe you didn't tell me." So, I did what I know how to do as a short person in a confrontation with a tall person: I stepped into his space.

I held up both hands and in a low, deep voice said, "Enough. How dare you speak to my husband like that. You breezed in without reading the chart and put your ungloved germ-covered hospital hands into Rockey's gaping wound. So, who put who at risk here? Rockey and I both stated at least four times today that he has Hep C. If your hospital didn't note that on his chart, that is certainly no fault of Rockey's." I looked at the computer screen. "Oh look. It says it right there in his chart. If anyone owes an apology here, it's you, Doc."

I took Rockey's good hand in mine as a sign of solidarity and looked at Rock. He said very softly to Cocky Doc, "Get out." As the door swished shut Rock looked at me and said, "What the hell? Did I deserve that?"

I said, "No way. It was unprofessional and everyone has been wearing gloves when touching a patient since about 1982. You always state your Hep-C status before anyone touches you. I heard you tell the nurses, and I told the EMTs. He didn't read your chart before he started. You didn't do anything wrong, Rock. He was out of line. He was so busy showing off, he forgot to do his job."

Rock looked at Lori and asked, "What say you, Lori?"

She shook her head and said, "That was crazy, and Mag is right. You didn't do anything wrong."

"Well, I don't care how good he is, I don't think I want that ass to be my doctor for this thing."

Lori offered, "I have a good friend who is the head of Orthopedics at one of the clinics, I could call him. He'd be happy to offer a suggestion."

I looked at Rock and said, "Your hand, your choice, Rock. What do you think?"

He considered it for a moment and looked at Lori and said, "Call your guy, please."

While Lori walked off talking into her phone, I looked out the door and told Rock that Cocky Doc was on the phone, and he looked worried. We both had a little giggle at that idea and just then the doctor turned and walked back into the room. His demeanor was very different than his first approach, and he looked at me and said, "I'm sorry. I overreacted and I should never have talked like that."

I said, "Don't apologize to me. He's your patient."

He turned to Rock and said the same words, and Rock said, "I'm not sure I want you to fix my hand." The doctor looked surprised and even a bit humbled, and Lori walked back in and nodded to Rockey. Rock asked the doctor to "Give us a minute, will you?" and Cocky Doc exited the room.

Lori laid out her findings, which included the other hand doctor in town as well as some scheduling issues, meaning Rockey's reconstruction surgery would be delayed by at least a week. He thought about that for a minute and Cocky Doc came back. He looked at me and started to speak, and I pointed at Rock and said, "Your patient." He turned his attention to Rockey, apologized again and made the pitch for his excellent skills.

Rock looked at me and I spread my hands indicating it was his call, and he said slowly and in his soft voice, "When would you do the surgery?"

"First thing Monday," the doctor said.

I lowered my chin and raised my eyebrows at Rock, communicating the way only people with a long history can do, and he looked at the doctor and said, "Okay, first thing Monday and I hope you're as good as you think you are."

The doctor looked relieved and said, "I'll do a great job for you."

Rock didn't miss a beat when he said, "I expect you will. Otherwise, it's her that you'll have to deal with. She's my voice and she takes that job seriously." He smiled a Rockey smile at me and then at the doctor as the doctor backed out of the room.

Lori, Rockey and I all sighed at having a resolution, and I went to look for the paperwork I'd need on Monday, and to determine whether I could take him home now. I told Lori I'd buy her dinner if she would grab something for us all and I'd swing by her place on our way home and pick it up. Rock gave her a peck on the cheek and a "Thanks, Lori!" as she bent down to hug him. The nurses rebandaged his messy hand and arm, gave him a shot of antibiotics and sent us off with more, as well as some painkillers, saying, "Don't uncover this or get it wet and we'll see you at 7:00 a.m. Monday."

While I waited with a lightly sedated Rockey in pre-op on Monday morning, Cocky Doc stopped in and took another look at his hand. He said, "This pinky finger looks a little dusky. I'll try to reattach it, but we may need to schedule another surgery to amputate it if it doesn't get good blood flow."

I looked at Rock and he made a slashing motion across his neck, and I addressed the doctor: "Rockey says take it now. He doesn't want another surgery."

The doctor's eyes slid from me to Rock and back again, and he gave a puzzled look and said, "Okay. I'll see you in there."

The surgery was expected to last about two hours, so I left the hospital to get some groceries and supplies for redressing his wound. While I was out, Cocky Doc called and said, "His little finger isn't pinking up the way I'd like to see. I don't think it will be functional. What do you want me do to?"

I told him Rockey and I had discussed it and Rock was not interested in trying to save it at the risk of having to undergo another surgery. "Take it off, please, if its survival is questionable."

He said, "Okay. I'll be wrapping up here in about fifteen minutes, then he'll go to recovery. You can see him there and, barring any complications, you should be able to take him home after lunch."

The surgery went well and was mostly dozens of stitches inside and on the outside. The saw had cut muscle, nerves, and tendons, so the doctor cautioned Rockey about regaining full use of the hand. Maybe because of his tolerance for pain, Rock was not terribly uncomfortable as he recovered, unless he inadvertently bumped it. It was covered in a very thick bandage, and he wore a sling for two weeks. As soon as they removed the stitches, he started physical therapy. Other than an occasional twinge in his absent pinky finger, he made a fabulous recovery. He was never able to wear a watch or his wedding ring again because both irritated the scar, and we agreed that Cocky Doc was, indeed, very good at his job.

Summer ended and elk season opened. It was Rockey's happy time of year. Elk hunting and baby giggles had lifted his spirits, so he was almost content as 2016 faded away.

Patches
2017

The new year in this house started with and maintained a feeling of dread after the results of the 2016 election. Both of us were guilty of this, but Rock became mildly obsessed with watching the news for hours, covering the ridiculous to the appalling actions of the newly elected goon. He gained a depth of understanding of our political culture and had speech been less of a struggle for him, we would have had more great conversations on the topics of the day. We had both always leaned far left politically and I was an avid reader of political issues. Rock was firm in his liberal beliefs but had never followed it all as closely as I had until this election season. It was a bit like watching a train wreck: you know you should look away; you know you can't fix it and you know watching will only make you feel worse. And yet we persisted, feeding our fears for our country every day. With the announcements of the Cabinet picks, the Muslim ban or the lessening of Environmental regulations, Rock yelled at the TV. We both felt strongly about the sacredness of public lands and strong environmental policies. One day, Rock was helping Andi build a Lego tower and I heard him say, "If we're not careful sweetie, this guy will put towers and mines in every wilderness we love." Andi said, "We love *wild-O-ness*, don't we, Papa? We should be careful."

Rockey began drawing plans for a horse run-in to create some shelter in their hot summer pasture. I asked him about cutting the wood and whether he felt ready to run a saw again. He held up his left hand with its stubby pinky finger and said, "I think this message is clear. My sawing days are over. I'll do all the measuring and stacking and get one of the guys to do the cuts." He seemed to accept this new adjustment without rancor or sadness and went back to his measuring and drawing. Rock had always been a thrifty guy and had, over the years, saved many board feet of lumber left over from various projects. He said with a grin, "I have almost enough cedar in my board pile to build the whole thing. There are some short pieces that I can use on the far side, if you don't mind some piece work that no one will see. I also have enough of that green metal roofing to cover it. Are you okay with that even though it won't match the barns?" I was ecstatic to be getting this shelter and couldn't have cared less about a green roof and some short boards.

"You bet I'm okay with that. What can I do to help?" I said and raised my eyebrows to make a big-eyed look. We had spent years on the farm doing big and small construction projects successfully together. But as Rock's motor skills began to dim, he often knocked into me with boards or other things and reacted with anger if he inadvertently hurt me. He wasn't mad at me, but the anger always ruined the moment. We both acknowledged that his reaction was ass-backwards, but he wasn't able to not get mad and I wasn't okay with the yelling. That had made us reluctant to take on hard projects together, but I could help him set up and get the location ready, as long as we weren't occupying the same space while lifting heavy things. As I walked away, I wondered how he would be able to manage all the walking, all the bending, lifting, and twisting required to build a small shelter. I wasn't willing to dampen the mood with questions about practicality, so I kept them to myself.

This whole year went like this. Quiet efforts made toward forward motion. His cognizant skills continued to diminish almost imperceptibly unless he chose to engage in conversation longer than the typical two sentences. There were not gaping holes in his mental acuity, but he would make odd errors. His prowess with numbers and measuring were well known, but the measuring for this simple project got the best of him some days, and he was frustrated by the need to double check everything he measured and then discover mistakes. Sometimes when we sat together in the evenings, Rock watching TV and me playing scrabble or reading on my iPad, he would say something. Often, these sentences would have a couple words that went together, but the rest of the sentence would be unrelated or bizarre words. I never felt compelled to point out his mistake, so I would think for a minute, hoping to decipher what he meant. Most times when my response was delayed, he would wince and say, "That was word salad, wasn't it?" I'd issue a sigh of relief that he knew and nod in assent. He would usually laugh a little and say, "I have no idea what I meant to say."

Through all the weeks, Andi kept her scheduled visit at our house and Rockey would go over to Nick and Megan's on Saturday mornings to hang out with the kid. Megan worked on Saturdays, and I think Nick liked the idea of team-watching the child with his dad. Rock was still just nimble enough to be on the floor with Andi; there are scores of photos with the two of them wearing silly grins. The gift of the grandchild may have been the single most powerful reason for him to keep trying to live.

He made another trip to Fort Peck for fishing that summer and it was to be his last. He took his friend Dave from Big Sky along; I took Dave aside before they left. I asked him to watch over Rock, emphasizing that if Rockey went over the side, don't wait around. "Something robbed him of his ability to swim. I'm pretty sure he'd sink like a stone, so be quick about saving him. With all the set-up chores, just butt right in and help him with anything that needs doing." Dave and Rock had been friends for twenty years, but Dave was a passive fellow, and I could picture him standing by, waiting to be asked for help. I had fried some chicken and made a giant bowl of potato salad to send along, and I packed it into the fridge in the RV. Once more, I watched him drive away with the impossibly long rig and hoped that all would go well, glad he was still willing to try to do the hard stuff.

Sprinkled throughout this year that we valiantly tried to fill with normal pleasures and pursuits was Rockey's growing insistence that someone somewhere had a magic bullet, through some miraculous surgery, that would stop the ravages happening to his body and return him to his formidable self. In his mind he had successfully erased Parkinson's as the primary thief of his physicality. Meanwhile, I was losing patience with this crazy chase he was on.

Rockey and Dave returned after two days of fishing, earlier than they planned. Rock called once he got a cell signal and told me they were on their way, saying he had run aground and bent the propeller on the boat. When he stepped through the door after he and Dave had unhooked the boat, plugged in the RV and Dave had headed up the canyon to his house, I had enough of a glimpse of Rock's face to know that something bigger than a bent propeller had chased them home. I figured he would tell me the story when he was ready. It took a few days, but he finally did.

They were on the big lake fishing for walleye and had driven the boat to an island for a bathroom break. Off the boat, they went their separate ways. The ground was a mix of sand and rocks, and Rock lost his balance and fell. He was on a small downslope when he fell with his head pointed down the little hill and couldn't right himself. He struggled, too humiliated to call out for help. By the time he got himself turned around and was able to stand, he was sweaty, tired and a little bit panicked. That was it. They packed up that night and headed home the next morning. I don't think he meant for that to be his last fishing trip, but it turned out that even though he would plan several more trips in the next two years, he always found a reason to cancel and never went back to Fort Peck.

But Rock continued to prepare for his horse shelter project. I helped gather his supplies and move them down to the site for the lean-to. He had become cranky again and was difficult enough to be around without having something stupid devolve into a yelling and throwing fit, so I helped when I could while staying out of his circle of anger. His body wouldn't cooperate with the demands of the construction project, and he finally called a younger friend named Brad to help.

Brad was strong, fast and an excellent carpenter, and together they made quick work of the shed. Brad was a Rockey devotee. He was in his late thirties and perpetually in trouble with the law for DUIs and escalating petty crimes. When he used meth, he was out of control. He was always straight when he came to see us. He was a "sand war" veteran—his words, not mine—and suffered from PTSD. He came from an eastern state where he was no longer allowed to visit because of a warrant for his arrest. That wasn't a problem as long as his beloved dad could come here for visits. The year before this building project, his dad was diagnosed with cancer and died soon after the diagnosis. Brad was devastated. He sought Rockey out more often in the months following his dad's death, and I told Rock to be aware that Brad needed his steady friendship now more than ever. They fished and hunted. Some days, Brad stopped in at dinnertime and always seemed happy to be invited to eat with us. He got sober for a long time, and I think hanging with us, with Rockey, was a safe place to distance himself from his old habits. No matter what trouble he had gotten into, Rock always offered him a safe place to land and unconditional friendship.

It seemed that at least once a year, we had reason to clash over the fact that Rockey had neglected to include my name on the deed to the farm. This year, there was an issue with the property taxes, and it required a visit to the courthouse. The courthouse had become a nearly impossible destination for Rock because it was a long walk from any parking spot, and there were stairs. Lots of stairs.

Rockey opened the notice and tossed it to me across the counter saying, "You want to go down there and straighten this out, please?"

I read the letter, tossed it back and said, "I'd be happy to, but you seem to have forgotten that I'm not listed as a property owner. I have as much right to fix this as Hay Ray" (a local barfly). "If you had changed it, I could help, but alas, I'm just the housekeeper."

That was more than I should have said, and he blew up. The last thing I heard as I walked out the door was, "I did everything, and you did nothing. I made this … blah, blah, blah." There was never a resolution to this issue, and it festered in my heart and in my mind.

Journal Entry

9/28/17

There are some things I can't get over. The shock and betrayal of not having my name included on so many documents is still bright and hot on my heart. That I was told that I "forced him to marry me" is another stunner that never dims. The way these moments of mistrust and disrespect have crept into and eroded my identity are so disappointing to me. I question my own ability to judge people and their truths. How could I have ignored early signs of this lack of equality he views me with? How did I manage to overlook his reticence to see me as a partner, his efforts to exclude me from marital property or just the decency one might expect to receive after being a good other half? Instead of growing warmer with the years of being together, his diseases have made these traits more obvious or more difficult for him to hide.

I now see I wait for the snappish retort, the martyr-ish statement or the outright contempt toward my opinions and thoughts. It has made me careful with my words and I use my words less often. Silence feels like my safest place. I am sorry to admit that I am afraid of him. I think he would hurt me. I think he would kill the dogs or my horses to spite me, if he were angry enough. I truly believe he would throw me out and spend the next day insuring I had no access to anything—not that I have much now.

I am ashamed to admit that I have allowed this exclusion from information and access and equal ownership. I allowed myself to be set down or beneath. I was always quick to judge older women who found themselves in this position—one with little knowledge of where the finances stood and limited access to those things.

I have allowed myself to be treated as a subordinate. That really pisses me off. I tiptoe because he's sleeping. I tiptoe because he's unable to deal with what's happening to him. I tiptoe because he seems unable to grasp ideas or conversations like he used to. I tiptoe because he's sad or mad or secretive. I feel like an intruder in my own home. I do not feel like I'm part of a team. I do not feel like he's on my side, or in my corner or that he has my back.

Over time, I have allowed all of this. It seems I've become less bright, less intense, less sure of myself in the world. I did not deserve to be excluded. I did not mean to become subordinate.

Every night we would go to bed and watch some TV together, always David Letterman until he retired and ruined my life. As Rock drifted off, I would take my pillow and move to the couch. The night terrors were an every night occurrence now, and I no longer waited to leave the bed until the yelling started. In the morning I would return to bed and we'd watch some morning news together and have some coffee. While I brushed my teeth, Rock would go to the kitchen, pour two cups of coffee with cream, and bring them to the bedroom. For every morning of our life together, he brought me coffee in bed. On this morning he had been bringing me morning coffee for 24 years. Recently, his hands curled awkwardly around the cups, and he had grown unsteady on his feet, spilling a little along the way. I never rose to help him, lest I infringe on something important to him. This day he tripped, and his cup flew into the air and rolled under the bed. My cup flipped onto the bed with its entire contents spilling onto the covers. He caught himself before falling and looked at me with the saddest eyes and said, "I guess I'm all done being the coffee guy." I got up and went to him, pulled off his coffee drenched t-shirt and grabbed a clean one. I said, "It's high time I got my skinny ass out of bed and did my part. We won't live enough years for me to catch up, but I'll be happy to be the coffee girl now." A small meaningful gesture that he had to abandon. I never minded the spilling but was deeply saddened that he had to give up one more thing that mattered to him. I put my arms around him once more trying to patch the hole of another loss.

A Different Kind of Wreckage
2018

It's safe to say the new year didn't dawn with joy. Maybe the grayness of winter affected our moods, or maybe it was because we tend to have an unmet expectation for the feeling of newness or a restart when January rolls around, but damn, the mid-winter blues had become a dreaded annual visitor.

Rockey seemed to have made a silent resolution, which was to get some surgery. By mid-January, we were sitting in an orthopedic surgeon's office in Billings, where Rock was making his pitch to get a hip replacement. The X-ray didn't show great joint damage from arthritis, but just enough to justify some new hardware. I have no doubt that Rock experienced daily pain in his back, legs, and joints, which he declared to the surgeon. The part left unsaid was that he had convinced himself that a new hip joint would enable him to walk with ease. It was the same old story and the same set of outrageous expectations. I tried to lead the doctor into asking Rockey what he hoped to gain from the surgery, but he didn't pick up my cues. So, with the expectation question unasked, they set a date for hip replacement surgery in mid-February at St Vincent's in Billings.

My concerns for seeking these surgeries weren't just because I didn't believe they would improve his physical abilities. I had no justification with my concerns but that did nothing to diminish them. I had a feeling of foreboding but didn't have any science to back me up. So, plans were made.

I was able to talk the doctor into keeping Rockey for a couple extra days after the new hip installation. Typically, they release joint replacement patients after a one-night stay in the hospital. I asked that Rock receive an extra forty-eight hours to ensure that he was able to rise from a chair or the bed without assistance, since he was already becoming weaker. I reminded Rockey that I too was aging and hauling him around had become too hard to do alone. I needed him to be strong enough to contribute to the effort. He had major objections to this request, but I insisted to the doctor and to Rockey that I was unwilling to risk injury to myself. I might have left the impression that I would be unavailable should he be released too soon. I felt like the bad guy once again. How dare I have concerns about my own safety?

I found someone to stay at the farm while we were gone, and a few days before we were scheduled to go to Billings, the weather report called for a big snowstorm that was expected to drop several feet of snow between Bozeman and Billings. Rather than driving in a snowstorm on Sunday, I moved our hotel reservation to include Saturday night. The surgery was to be early Monday morning. When we checked into the hotel late Saturday afternoon, the roads were still clear and dry, and Rock made a point to be pissy about coming a day early for my imaginary snowstorm. By 7:00 p.m. at least a half foot of snow had fallen, and I felt vindicated. Burning up a whole Sunday in a small hotel room with nowhere to go seemed a small inconvenience compared to a white-knuckle drive.

Rock was registered and checked in by 6:00 a.m. Because of the weather, I planned to wait to see him in recovery, then head for home in what would be a long and slow drive. He was in rough shape when I got to his room, with intense pain and an altered mind. The bandages on the incision bothered him, and he kept trying to remove them. He had the same delusion as other times, thinking he was a prisoner and yelling about being held against his will. The surgeon stopped in and told us both that the surgery had gone very well. Rockey said, "Well, I'm glad you think so. It feels like you used a chain saw to open me up."

I went to the bed to hug and kiss him, showed him his bag of extra clothes and phone charger. He was mad that I was leaving, and I told him again that he'd be doing a little rehab for just a couple days and then would come home. I made sure there was an order on file for plenty of pain meds and waited until they had given him some before I left.

The drive back was slow, but I set my tires in the ruts of the slow lane and stayed on the highway going 60 mph. The crazy drivers who refused to acknowledge the poor conditions dotted the ditches as I made my way slow and sure. Poor Rock was tangled up in his mind again. My phone rang often, and he was yelling about being a prisoner and the movement detection device on the bed proved it. I tried to tell him that they wanted to be sure he wasn't trying to get up without assistance. Nope. He didn't accept that explanation and quizzed me again and again about why he was in custody.

Each morning from home, I checked with the nurses and was told he was doing well with the rehab. It was his mind that was creating problems. Lucky for me, Nick offered to pick him up as the roads were still in rough shape. I had expected him home on Thursday, but because his anxiety was escalating, I asked them to release him Wednesday. When he got home, into his favorite chair, he became less shrill and less angry. His mind was still altered, and he couldn't remember from one moment to the next where he had been and why. This time, it was nine days until his mind returned to something more normal.

For at least the first year after the hip replacement, I think Rockey would have said it was a success. He said he had less pain in his joint and went to physical therapy twice a week for a few months. He used his walking sticks to help with his balance as he tried to walk from the house to the shop, even though he would complain of muscle soreness after those excursions. The truth was his walking continued to deteriorate and he didn't have the gains from the surgery he was hoping for.

I had found an unusual cart while snooping around online one day. This little beauty could be custom made, which was a huge plus because of Rockey's height. It used four fat bicycle tires and electric bicycle batteries for power and the video showed it going through snow and up mountain trails maintaining an adequate speed of 12 mph with a range of ten to twenty miles per charge on the batteries. The cart was made in Utah so we could easily make a trip to test-drive one. It was also affordable at less than $5,000. Other carts I had found with off-road capabilities were often priced out of reach at $30,000. I thought it might be the perfect answer to give Rock more freedom of movement. I did the research, had pictures and a video, and made my pitch, but Rockey wouldn't even consider it. It was certainly his decision to make, but I always felt that his refusal to even try one of these machines was a self-defeating choice for him. It made me sad that he couldn't find a way to accept it.

By summer, he was fully recovered and made himself bale the ten acres of hay we had someone cut. The big alfalfa field was now leased by a local hay producer who cut and baled it on shares with us. Getting in and out of the tractor was more of a challenge every year, but the satisfaction of doing the work made it worth it to Rock. In the past year, he started to verbalize his feelings of worthlessness more often, so any task that was doable was important. After the hay was cut, my friend Nancy and I would use the hayfields to work our dogs on sheep-herding skills. I always asked Rockey for help dragging us around to set up markers and panels for the courses we made. We'd load our gear in his Ranger and he was happy to haul us around and drop us and the equipment around the big fields. Even though I was competent at most of the tasks around the farm, I tried to keep a running list of small projects to ask for Rock's help with. It pleased him to have jobs to do, but it wasn't quite enough to keep him from feeling as if he was a burden. We often sat outside in the evenings, and it was one of the few times we still had substantial conversations. It still took him a long time to form words, and he used them sparingly, but he began to talk more often about suicide. He couldn't find any way to make peace with his failing body and his sluggish mind. He was aware that his mental acuity was dimming rapidly, and it scared him almost as much as his loss of physicality.

He would become weepy on the nights we talked like this, and it was heartbreaking for us both. I mostly just listened to his soft speech and tried to hug away his tears. I don't think there was much possible comfort for Rockey in those days, but I tried my best to be who he needed me to be for these talks. I never offered advice or discouragement. I just let him talk. One night after we'd had one of these sad, sad conversations, I heard the notification sound on my phone. I could see Rockey texting and just assumed he was chatting with one of the kids. When I checked the message, it was from Rock. I had one more trip to the pasture to get the horses back in off the grass, so I took my phone and set off to get the fat ponies in.

Summer waned, and elk season came around again and buoyed Rockey's spirits. I was taking my horse Louie once a week or so to a young horse trainer nearby to help get a little finishing on some specific skills. It was a vaguely peaceful moment in time for both Rock and me. One sunny Sunday in October, my friend Lori picked me and Louie up with her horse trailer and we went up the canyon and into the buffer zone of Yellowstone Park for one last sunny horse ride before winter settled in. The day was as perfect as a mountain girl could hope for. Clear blue skies, no wind, and a long-sleeved shirt kind of day. It was my first mountain ride on Louie, and he traveled like he was born to do this trail on this day.

Lori was riding her good old horse Stinky, who never made any mistakes. We went ten miles on a southern-exposure dry trail with good footing, and as we got closer to the end, I thought it was the best day on horseback I'd had in a very long time. Lori wanted to cut through the woods on our return to the trailhead, and in the shade, the frosty nights had created a bit of ice. I had cautioned her earlier that we'd best stay out of the trees if we wanted to avoid icy footing.

I watched as Stinky set his feet and slid down a short but steep little hill covered with ice. I called out to Lori, "I'm not sure Louie can handle a slide like that, I'm going to hop off." I swung easily out of the saddle, took two steps and my feet flew out from under me like a cartoon kind of ice fall. I yelped and said, "I'm okay," and I tried to stand. I fell back to the ground and said to Lori, "Oh no. Not okay. It's not okay. I can't get up. My right leg doesn't work." I let go of the reins and Louie walked off toward Lori and Stinky. I laid on my left side with my good leg on the ground and found if I stacked the right leg by pulling on my jeans to move it, I didn't have much pain.

Lori had gotten off, and she said, "What do you want me to do?"

"I can't walk, and I can't get back on, so you'll have to go get help."

She held out her hand and said, "Gimme your phone."

"Why?" I asked. She said hers was dead and she would call. I said, "Oh no. There's no signal for almost twenty miles. You'll have to either use a land line at the 320 Ranch or go to the old Half Moon Saloon, that's where cell phones start to work again."

"Shit," she said.

"It's okay. Just give me all the jackets and catch Louie and take him out with you." I had more wilderness experience than Lori, but she was one of the best horsewomen I knew, so I had no doubts she'd get out and bring help, plus we were only about a mile and a half from the parking lot.

She draped the jackets over me and with a quick look down at me, she said, "I'll be back as quick as I can."

I could see Stinky's shiny bay coat as they disappeared into the trees, and I looked up to see the position of the sun and checked the time: 3:45 p.m. I figured I'd never be rescued before the sun went down and I shivered, knowing I was going to get real cold. For the moment, I was comfortable as long as I didn't try to move my right leg, but the ground was icy where I fell and I thought once the adrenaline wore off, I might be pretty chilly. My bad leg was resting with no pressure, but I was laying on my long-ruined left shoulder. I had to laugh out loud as it was surely a *what-the-fuck* moment. It dawned on me almost right away that I was lying immobile in bear country in late October, and Lori had ridden off with my bear spray. I laughed again. I was laying right in the trail and would have been a surprise to any riders coming around that tree to my left. Not wanting to cause anyone a wreck, I tried to move off the trail. That effort lasted only a few seconds until I realized that dragging my bad leg was going to bring on some pain fast. So, I settled in to wait. A little squirrel hopped up on a log not far from me and started chittering loudly at my intrusion. I was laying with pinecones scattered all about, and I grabbed one and started peeling off the seeds and tossing them to my noisy visitor. Nothing. He didn't even pick up a seed. He just kept up his alarm calls.

I think it was about ninety minutes before I heard hooves on the trail coming in from the west, the direction that rescue people would start coming from. I heard Lori call out, and I answered her, remembering that I was not on the trail because we had been looking for it when I fell, so she needed to hear me to locate me. After making sure I was still all right, she gave me the scoop. "First, I ran into a couple leaving the parking lot and I gave them Rock's number and told them to call him and tell him you were in a wreck but were okay. Then a state trooper drove by, so I flagged him down and he called the park rangers and an ambulance for the rescue." She said with excitement, "Can you believe how lucky we are that the trooper was going by? He's standing by the trailer now keeping Louie calm, because he went nuts when I rode away. The rescue guys and the EMTs will arrive in about an hour. Are you warm enough? The trooper gave me this radio so I can guide them in and, oh Jesus! I rode away with the bear spray, I'm so sorry."

I laughed at her motormouth and said, "It's okay. I wasn't scared. You should keep it because you're riding through all those willows by the water."

She walked over to her horse and dug a big silk scarf out of the saddlebag and wrapped it around my neck. It felt nice and warmed me right away and it smelled like Lori. She took my face in her hands and said, "They're on the way, Maggie. You'll be heading out of here in no time. Are you still okay?"

I smiled and said, "I am!"

She had nothing else to give me except a smile as she mounted up and said, "I better go look for them so they can find you. Be back as soon as I can."

Once again, I watched Stinky's shiny coat get swallowed by the trees and brush. I took a selfie as the day started to dim—one of my face and one of my feet. I suppose I was in shock because the next thing I remember was a rugged-looking guy, smiling broadly and striding along with three other rescuers. They wasted no time and Rugged Man knelt beside me, asking how I was doing. A woman knelt down and told me she was a paramedic and checked my breathing and heart rate. She said, "Good job, Maggie, you're doing great." Someone asked what I needed most, and I said, "I'm really getting cold." They asked what time I laid down and I told them, and they laughed and said, "OOOh, tough girl! It's been almost three hours." Somebody took out a huge wool hat and pulled it down on my head, then put my hands in the warmest mittens I've ever felt.

Two guys were working on getting a tarp and some blankets under me and Rugged Man said, "Sorry, I have to cut your boots off."

I said, "No, no you don't, they're easy, just pull them off."

He cocked his head. "I think that will hurt your leg."

I shook my head "I promise I'll tell you if it hurts, but I'm sure you can pull these boots right off."

He carefully placed his hands and pulled the boots easily off my feet. I smiled at him. Then he said, "Well, I for sure have to cut those jeans off."

I answered, "Yes, you do because I am not trying to lift this butt up for you."

Pants off, I could hear the familiar hushed tones of medical people not wanting to alarm the patient. By now, whoever was in charge of the blankets and getting me on the litter was ready for the next step. "Okay Maggie, we have to lift you up to get the blankets under you and while we do that, these guys will slide the litter under you. We'll move as fast as we can and do everything possible not to hurt you."

I looked around and realized there were lots more rescuers, a total of ten now, and boom, they had me up, wrapped and set back down before I could even worry about it. The burrito-fashioned blankets felt so wonderful. I felt such gratitude, and then the woman EMT said, "That's not the blankets, I just gave you some morphine."

Rugged Guy moved in close and said, "It's going to be dark soon. You have about two minutes to decide whether you want a helicopter."

I asked, "Do you think they take Medicare?" We all snorted a little laugh and I said, "Sorry guys, it's all on you to get me out."

"No worries," he said. "We live for this stuff. How much do you weigh, Maggie?"

"About one hundred and forty," I answered.

Faint applause rippled in the air, and he said, "We're always grateful for the little people."

Then like some backcountry choreography, I was in the air, and we were heading through the trees. As we traveled, I had my right hand resting on my inner thigh and it felt weird. I chose this moment to throw the blankets and look at my leg. The skin wasn't broken, but a bone was going sideways and causing the skin to tent. I started swearing loudly and saying, "Oh Jesus, oh goddammit, why did I look at that?"

Rugged Man stopped the carriers and leaned into my face while he wrapped the blankets around me again. He said, "Maggie, seeing it doesn't change what's happened. Your femur is broken and we're going to get you to a hospital as fast as we can and you're going to be all right. Right?" I stopped hollering, looked at his face, nodded and they resumed carrying.

There were three people on each side of the litter, at least two walking ahead and two more behind. It was full dark now and if I opened my eyes, I could see their headlamps bobbing and lighting their way. The two front walkers acted as the spotters for the ones carrying me. They would call out things in the trail: "Big rock, right front." "Low stump, left side." With each call, the carriers would so gently lift me to avoid getting hooked or bumping any obstacles. I never once felt jostled or rocked or anything but perfectly safe. Every so often, someone would gently peel the blankets away from my face, look in my eyes intently and say, "Are you still doing okay, Maggie?" I was in and out of consciousness and can just barely remember hearing their boots cross the foot bridges close to the parking lot.

Then I was in the ambulance and those guys were incredibly kind as well. I asked where they were from and one responded, "We're from Hebgen Lake. We are the bus on call for park emergencies tonight."

I uttered a "Wow!" Hebgen sounded so far away.

"We'll be taking you to Idaho Falls tonight, if that's okay."

I said, "Oh no. Can't you take me to Bozeman? Idaho Falls would be so hard on Rockey. My husband is disabled, and Idaho Falls is so far for him to drive. We live in Gateway."

He said, "Sure, we'll take you to Bozeman. Idaho Falls is the Trauma Center the Park usually uses, that's all." He banged on the noisy metal sides and said, "We're going to Bozeman." And the driver pulled out onto the highway for the two-hour drive. The guy riding with me checked my heart and blood pressure and gave me some more morphine. The next thing I knew I came to in a room I recognized as Bozeman Health, and Rockey was sitting in a chair next to my bed crying hard. I saw Nick standing off to the side of the room.

I reached out and took Rock's hand and said, "Oh honey, it's okay. I'm going to be okay. Don't be worried now."

"I've been so scared. I didn't know what happened and they called so long ago, and I didn't know where you were." The words tumbled out of his mouth as he sobbed.

Nick said something like, "Your leg is blown up. I saw the X-ray."

I took a deep breath and patted Rock's hand some more and said, "Nothing more will happen tonight. You should let Nick take you home. Did you feed the dogs?"

"No. I forgot. But I called Kath and she's coming to help. She's coming to take care of you," he said, trying to look hopeful.

I looked at him and said, "See, now you've got work to do. Lori probably has all my stuff and I'm sure she'll bring you my phone and stuff tomorrow. Did you have any supper?" He shook his head. I looked at Nick and said, "Maybe you can drive through someplace on the way home and get him some food, eh?" I felt my drugged head becoming unable to guide the Goertz boys any longer and I said, "I'm pretty drugged up, fellas. I think that's all the talking I can do. You watch over your dad, Nick. Thanks for bringing him. We'll figure it all out tomorrow, Rock. Don't forget to feed the dogs." I kissed Rock's hand and fell off the world.

Bad Break
Late October 2018

When I woke Monday morning, it was to nurses turning on bright lights, taking blood pressure readings and blood samples, and checking the output from my catheter.

"When did you do that?" I asked.

"They put it in when you were in the ER," they said. The nurses kept asking me to put a number on my pain and I knew the frown-faced chart by heart from all Rockey's hospital experiences.

"It's a two if I don't move, but I can get it up to a five or six pretty easily. But I can't move the leg at all."

"Hasn't anyone told you? You are not to try to get up or move without assistance, Maggie."

I smiled and nodded and said, "Yeah, I didn't even need to be told. I already know this leg doesn't work."

She softened a little and said, "We all heard about the rescue. Pretty incredible. Were you scared lying alone in the forest?"

I made my lips into a flat line and shook my head, saying, "I wasn't scared at all. I'd like to think it's just my fearless nature, but

I was probably in shock. I knew my friend would bring some help. I was more worried about how cold I was going to get when the sun set. The ground was frozen where I fell."

"Were you wearing warm clothes? Did you fall off your horse?" she asked.

I snorted a little laugh and said, "Nope. My good horse was just standing there. I took two steps and slipped on the ice, my feet flew up in the air and I landed on a pointy rock right where the break is. It was a nice, sunny fall day, but I had on a long-sleeved shirt and vest, with a heavy fleece jacket tied on my saddle. I wasn't terribly cold until about a half hour before they found me."

"That's what I wondered," she started to say, and then she was paged. "I'll be back," she said over her shoulder as she hurried out the door.

I slept on and off all morning and woke once to find Rockey and Lori in the room. It dawned on my foggy mind that he needed help to get here. My worried man did his best to smile at me when I awoke and even through the drug haze, my heart went out to him. His smile was trembling, and his eyes looked so scared.

I took his hands in mine and said, "Are you doing okay, Rock?"

Tears filled his eyes, and he squeezed my hands hard and said in his whispery voice, "No. No, I'm not okay. I'm so worried about you." Pause. "And me. I don't know how to do anything, Mag."

A few tears slid down my face and I said, "We'll be all right. We're always all right, Rock."

He paused a little too long and finally said, "Because of you. We're only all right because of you. I don't know what to do."

I gave him a dopey smile and said, "You're doing it right now … just what you should do. You have a bag of something there for me, you have a good traveling pal. You called Kath. When is she coming, by the way?"

"She's coming Wednesday, I think," he answered.

Lori was fussing around, straightening my supplies, and arranging stuff on my hospital tray. "Let's make this better so you can use it. I'll get it so you can reach everything." Shuffle, pick up, slide this over here; it was like watching a shell game with hospital trinkets as she got everything just so. She filled my hospital mug with ice water; I don't know where she found ice. She gave me my phone, lip goo—as I call all chapstick, a box of tissue and other sundries.

Rock set a bag on the chair and said, "All your stuff is in here."

This activity felt jangly to me, and while I appreciated the efforts, I just wanted everyone to stop moving and stop talking. I finally said, "Okay you two, thanks for worrying and thanks for bringing me some things. I took more drugs before you got here, and I think I have to sleep again. I'm okay, really. I don't know what happens next, but I'll call you when I find out. Kath will just swoop in and take care of everything, Rock. Just let her do that. Lori will get you home. Right?"

Lori slipped her arm through Rock's and said, "Yup. I'm going to take Rockey home and get something to eat set up so it's easy for him to warm up." She winked at me. "I'll check the ponies and make sure the dog food is ready for Rock to feed later."

I gave a sleepy thumbs up and blew kisses at them and said, "Thanks!"

Later in the day (I recall it as mid-afternoon) a nurse came in and I was having some intense pain. He looked at my chart and said, "Is the Oxy working for you?"

I nodded and said, "This is the first big pain I've had."

He read some more and said, "You had a fair amount of morphine on board when you got in this room last night. That probably helped you until just now. Let's see if we can knock that pain down." He gave me a pill and a glass of water.

By the time he came back to my room, less than a half hour, I had thrown up. He gave me another Oxy, and the same thing happened. He asked, "Have you had trouble taking this before?"

I was starting to feel cranky about everything, and I said, "No. I've never had any trouble with anything, except Amoxicillin, but I've never been injured this badly either."

"What happened with Amoxicillin?" he asked.

"Anaphylactic shock," I replied. "It should be on my chart. The ambulance brought me here that day."

He opened the computer and scrolled for a bit, then his eyes widened, and he said, "Whoa! That was serious."

I just said, "Yup, pretty serious."

"Well, we need to try something else for your pain now."

I was getting impatient with throwing up and still hurting badly. I said, "No. Are you guys starving me because surgery is scheduled?"

He looked puzzled and said, "Your surgery isn't until Wednesday. No, we're not worried about you eating right now."

"Then I should get some food. What day is this?" He told me it was Monday. I shook my head and said, "I have only eaten an apple since Saturday night. We left on the ride Sunday morning. I had an apple for lunch and nothing since. If you'd give me some food, I could probably handle the narcotics better." He handed me a menu for the cafeteria and told me to pick anything. "I don't have my glasses, so I'd just have a grilled cheese and maybe some chips, not those creepy Sun Chips either."

He laughed and said, "I'll order it for you."

Then I said, "Wednesday surgery is not okay with me. Why so long? Shouldn't we be hurrying?"

He looked surprised and said, "Let me go find out more about that."

He returned with at least three other nurses, and one introduced herself and said she was the charge nurse. "Your surgery is on the schedule for 1:00 p.m. Wednesday. The surgeon is booked solid."

All my years of advocacy on behalf of Rockey served me now.

"No. I don't care if they're booked. Somebody needs to reschedule an elective surgery and take care of this emergency." I rolled back the covers and even I was surprised to see how bruised my thigh was. "I'm not here so I can ski better or get back to my climbing hobby. I need this to get fixed so I can walk again. We need to change that surgery time."

She shook her head, saying, "I can't make that decision."

I said, "I understand. I want to talk to whoever can make the decision. While I wait for that to happen, I really need to eat something. I'm feeling poorly right now and I'm sure eating will help."

Someone brought the grilled cheese and not Sun Chips. I felt better immediately and had no more trouble keeping the painkillers down. I dozed some and awoke again to my room filling up with people. Front and center stood an incredibly tall man with a doctor's coat over a hoody and soft worn jeans. To his right stood a nurse with Scandinavian, white-blond hair, and bright blue eyes. She was silent as he spoke.

"I'm Dr. G and I'm going be your surgeon. I understand you're not happy about the schedule."

I said, "Nice to meet you. No, I'm not happy about it at all. We should be wheeling into surgery right now, I say."

He scowled a little and asked, "Didn't they ask you if you wanted to go to Billings? I told them I was booked solid."

I replied, "I don't remember anyone asking and I probably would have said yes. This place has a reputation for poor customer service and at this moment, I can see why. You can't just throw me into the schedule over a long lunch break. This is an emergency. Elective surgeries get bumped all the time for emergencies. Bump somebody. And if you're not going to do that, you better get me on a helicopter to Billings on the hospital's dime, because I'm not letting go of this. It's this hospital's mistake and they should not have accepted me as a patient if I wasn't going to get fixed. You need to fix my leg before Wednesday. Is that unreasonable logic?"

His face may have blushed a little and he looked a bit contrite as he said, "No, it's not unreasonable. I've moved my schedule around and you're having surgery at 8:00 a.m. tomorrow. Does that sound all right to you?"

"That sounds great. Are you good at what you do?"

He gave me a warm smile and chuckled, saying, "Yes. I am really good at what I do, and I can fix that leg. Someday, you'll have to tell me the story. I'll go over how we're going to fix it when I see you in the morning. Are we good now?"

I smiled and said, "Yeah, we're good." The blue-eyed nurse gave me a subtle thumbs up and winked and they turned and left my room as did the cadre of watchers.

The fabulous young man who had been my nurse that day looked at me, raised his eyebrows and said, "Wow. You kicked his ass."

I said "I did not. I was just saying the truth. This is an emergency situation and should be treated as such. That's all."

He laughed and said, "Yeah, but you still kicked his ass. He's kinda the king of hips and trauma orthopedics."

"He can still be king. I just want to get fixed before the thing grows back together crooked." My sweet nurse was endlessly entertained by my boldness, and I just let him enjoy it.

The anesthesiologist stopped in shortly after, explained what she would be doing and asked if I had any questions. I bluntly told her, "I've only had anesthesia twice and I can tell you, I am a puker. Violent puker. If you can do anything to fix that, you'd be my hero."

She smiled and said, "Piece o' cake. I'll give you an epidural and you'll wake up like nothing happened. It's good you told me because I have an easy remedy for that." I had total confidence in the tiny sprite doctor.

After she left, I was pushing my hair out of face and snagged a twig and a couple of pine needles out of it. I said to the sweet nurse, "Hey, any way you can get me a hairbrush and a toothbrush? No mirror though. I don't want to see how bad I look after two days of no hairbrush or toothbrush. I sure could use some grooming aids. Both are missing from the bag Rock brought, but I'm not going to point it out to him."

"I'll see what I can find," he said.

As promised, Dr. G stopped into the room where I was being prepped for surgery in the morning. He talked about a rod and nails and other particulars that I wouldn't remember. He asked, "Are you nervous?"

"I sure am. I've never been hurt this bad before. Never stayed in a hospital. Just make it so I can walk."

He patted my leg, smiled and said, "Oh, it will be way better than that. I'll see you after."

When I woke up again, back in my room, I felt pretty darn good. No nausea and no pain, not then anyway. The surgeon stopped in and repeated the hardware he had used and other things he found when he saw my shattered femur. Once again, I forgot everything he said when he left the room. I slept for a few hours and when I woke up, I started talking about going home. I wanted them to release me the next day, Wednesday. A nurse told me that a physical therapy person would be by later and see how I was able to get around with a walker. Friends had been popping in and more than one of them brought me a 16-ounce vanilla latte with three shots and half the vanilla. That was a little bit of heaven for me.

The PT lady came in, and she scared me. She was very matter-of-fact and asked me to lift my broken leg. I tried and then I tried again. When nothing happened, and she saw the look of panic on my face, she said, "Oh, you weren't really supposed to be able to move it. Don't feel bad. Nobody can do that. I'm getting a walker brought to this room and I'm going to show you how to use it. Do not put any weight on your broken leg. You can touch the toe down for balance, but absolutely no weight on it. You're going to follow me to a physical therapy room and we're going to see how you do."

I passed the test and arranged with Rockey to have a neighbor with a low-riding SUV pick me up after lunch on Thursday. Rockey and Kathy stood beside the SUV as I struggled to get out. They both reached for me, and I said, "I got this," as I hopped to the steps. I headed for one of the big recliners and kind of dropped into it, hitting the button to raise the leg rest. They were scurrying about, gathering things I might need or want.

It didn't take long to realize that the big recliner was not going to work as my home base for the next eight weeks. It was very uncomfortable on my newly reconstructed metal carrying hip as I hobbled into the room we called The Porch/Dumpster Room and took the back cushions off the couch and tossed them aside. I gingerly sat and Kathy lifted my legs while I twisted my body and got nestled into a sitting position with my legs stretched out. We fiddled around with pillows under my legs until we found the right mix. I was happy and physically comfortable in my nest, the spot I would stay for the next eight weeks. With windows on three sides, the spectacular views of surrounding ranches were bound to be good for the days when my spirits were low. I worried about the weeks of gray winter skies in my future and vowed to try to keep a positive outlook.

Rockey seemed a little lost, but better to be home with two strong-willed sisters than to be alone in this house. As I expected, Kathy just took care of everything. More pillows, less pillows, something to eat, something for Rock to eat, feed the dogs; the list was endless, and she never seemed to stop moving. I made a calendar that looked as if it had been made by a child and marked off the days when I could quit taking blood thinners, quit wearing those awful compression stockings, staples out and other important dates for recovery. When I started writing this chapter, I called Kathy and asked her what it was like. She said, "You were scared and in great pain. You had to take narcotics, so you were mad and swore a lot. And we all got through it." She's such a talker.

But her short version was correct. Altogether, she took care of me and Rockey for five weeks. My old friend Karen came in for two weeks. At six weeks, with some salesmanship, I was able to weasel permission to start bearing weight on the bad leg and everyone could go home. Were it not for Kathy and Karen, my outcome would have been far more lifechanging and my gratitude to them both runs deep.

More Crazy
2019

One of the things about my broken leg that caused Rockey trouble was having to postpone another hip replacement. During my convalescence, he asked at least weekly when he could schedule it. In January, I finally said, "Here's the deal. You can have it whenever you want. But I cannot be the one taking care of you for at least a year. I can't lift, I can't do any of the things you'll need help with. I suggest you go into a rehab facility right after the surgery and stay for a week or so, until you can move around better. So have it done as soon as you want, if you understand that I can't be your person for this one. I am unwilling to compromise my own healing and this leg is going to be fragile for a long time. Sorry, dude."

He scowled and said, "Well, what does that mean, 'rehab facility'?"

"I don't know where they send people, Rock, but I know plenty of old people don't have someone to help after these surgeries and they go someplace until they get strong enough to manage on their own. Ask them where they send people."

He snorted and said, "I wouldn't remember for two minutes after they told me. Would you talk to them about it, please?"

I said, "Sure. When you call to schedule, give the scheduler my phone number and have her call me. I'll find out what the options are."

I had to go into the orthopedic office every few weeks for X-rays of my leg. By late January, my doctor was concerned about the healing. He had me follow him into his office and brought up all the X-rays, including the ones from the day of the fall, which I had never seen. I was surprised at the image of the wreckage.

I exhaled loudly and he said, "What?"

I said, "I slipped and fell on the ice. I didn't get hit by a car or tumble off a cliff. I can't believe there was so much damage from something so small."

"Just the perfect impact to blow it up," he said. Then he showed me the first image after surgery and the one taken that day, three months after. There was a space between the broken ends that he left to compensate for the shortening of the leg as it healed. He pointed at the space and said, "See here. It isn't filling in. It's called a nonunion. We should have seen bone growth here by now. I need to get back in there and fix it. Your leg is only held together by all these screws. It isn't strong enough to withstand any trauma."

I said, "Wait. Wait. Wait. Why now? Why can't we give it a little more time? Why isn't it healing?"

He said, "Remember when I told you I left a space so your leg wouldn't be shorter? Well, I was probably too aggressive with the space, and it isn't going to join the other part. It happens. Not often, but it happens."

I thought for a minute and replied, "Okay. I'll agree to a second surgery, but we have to wait. You met Rockey, right?" He nodded. "He could hardly manage the first surgery I had, if I do another right now, he'll be a basket case. Plus, he's going to have his second hip replacement. I have no one I can ask for help. I used all that up. Can you give me three months? I promise that if it is still a nonunion by April 30th, I'll agree to the second surgery."

He made a face and said, "All right. I'm pretty sure you're still going to need it. It's your life, but it isn't very fair that you have to compromise your own best interests because it's hard on someone else."

I shrugged and held up my hands and said, "It's what I have, though. Can you fix it so it heals?"

He quickly said, "Yes, I can. We'll put a bigger rod in, all the way to your knee this time and add some bigger nails. You want to listen in on a call with the wizard of broken femurs? I practiced with this guy in Florida, and he might be the best leg trauma guy in the country. I need you to sign a release saying it's all right to share the images and your information with him."

I didn't hesitate to say, "Sure I do." I signed the release, and he sent off the imaging and put us all on speaker phone. Mostly they talked in medical terms that didn't mean much to me, but I was impressed to hear him trying to find the best answers for the problems my case presented. I left feeling disappointed in a second surgery, but hopeful about a full-ish recovery.

Rockey arranged to have his hip replacement on February 11. This Billings orthopedics office now had a patient coordinator and she called to talk to me about the rehab options. She gave me names of a couple of places for hip surgery rehab that they preferred, and I promised to look them up and have Rockey decide. I took that opportunity to talk to her about my thoughts on Rockey seeking a surgical solution to the devastation caused by Parkinson's. I told her he had been turned down for surgeries in other clinics and asked her if they had a question on their intake form regarding the patient's expectations. She answered, "No," of course. Since she wasn't the doctor and he was already scheduled, I saw no reason to hold back. In my kindest voice, I told her I thought it was unethical for doctors to perform major surgeries on a man in Rockey's physical and mental condition. I told her that I believed that he was so ruined physically that he not only had little chance for his life to be enhanced by this surgery, but that it was far more likely it would be a detriment to his overall health. She was surprisingly open to this conversation and asked good questions, and we had a substantial talk about the issues of major surgery on patients like Rockey. I didn't, for one moment, think this conversation would change anything for Rockey or any other patients, but I was glad to finally say my piece about it to a medical person.

I found the rehab places on the internet and read up on each of them. I gave Rockey the virtual tour and told him what I thought. He chose the one that offered a private room and wouldn't make him eat in the dining room with other "guests." We agreed that he would stay there for one week and come home a total of nine days after his surgery. I was still too broken to be in a car long enough to get to Billings, so he had Nick take him and pick him up. I hoped Rock would gain ground in the rehab center, because I was in no shape to offer him any physical assistance when he returned home.

The surgeon called after they got out of the surgery and said everything went well. Rockey started phoning me about three hours later. He was mad about the pain, mad about being held against his will. "When are you coming to get me?" he asked. "Oh, that's a good excuse," he said when I told him I wasn't coming because of my own physical limitations. He had forgotten I still walked with a cane. These calls went on day and night from the hospital and then from the rehab center. He was hysterical and in much worse shape mentally than he had ever been post-op before.

I talked to the head nurse at the rehab center, and she confirmed that he was quite unhinged, "Much more so than most hip replacement patients we see. And he is becoming quite combative." By Friday morning, three days ahead of schedule, the rehab center called me and asked if I would take him home. "He is just too uncooperative for our facility to manage."

I called Nick with the news. He sighed and said, "Let me get the guys going on this job and I'll head over." I thanked him and texted him the address.

I opened the front door when I heard Nick's big diesel truck pull up. He came around to the passenger side to help a surprisingly frail Rockey out.

In less than a week, he had lost enough weight for it to be noticeable immediately. His color was pasty gray and he seemed unbelievably weak. Nick had to support him under his arms to help him up the three steps and into his big chair. As soon as Nick left, Rockey began to cry and said, "I can't believe you had me locked up again. Why would you do that, Margaret? That's the meanest thing that's ever happened to me and you did it." His voice rose to a blubbery shout at the end, and I just looked at him, at a complete loss as to how to respond.

Finally, I asked, "Did they send you home with any pain meds? Are you in pain now?" He was angry, pouty, and out of touch with reality. I felt a wave of hopelessness wash over me.

"Yes, there are meds in my kit, and what was the other question?" he said.

"Do you need some pain medication?" I asked.

"Yes, I do need some," he answered, sounding very much like a fitful child.

I leaned on my cane and walked to the bags that were on the floor. Bending was still something I couldn't do so I hooked the bag handle with my cane and dragged it over to a bench, sat down and retrieved his kit bag. I walked back and sat down near him and took out the packets to read the labels, found some pain stuff, squeezing one out of the foil for him. I got up, heading to the kitchen, and said, "I'll fix us something to eat." He stuck his hand out as I went by, and I stumbled then snapped at him, "You can't grab me. I can't stay upright if you grab me."

He looked at the cane and said, "What happened to you?"

I started walking again and said, "I fell on the ice," shaking my head. I knew when he scheduled this surgery that he had little regard for my condition, and I thought that forcing the rehab stay would have mitigated his physical needs upon his release. I was not prepared for the frail old man sitting in my living room, snarking at me for my use of a cane. I did the familiar self-talk that he wasn't responsible for his messed-up mind and inappropriate comments. The truth was, I was really pissed. My broken condition was an accident, and my recovery wasn't given a moment's thought and I found it beyond my skill set to offer him the compassion he seemed to think he deserved.

Months later, I would see that this surgery left Rockey quite broken. His mind was scrambled, he was afraid much of the time, he no longer knew what day it was. He went to PT two or three days most weeks for many months. I was also in PT during this time and, having different therapists, we sometimes ran into each other there.

He experienced an increase in the frequency of night terrors. I was still sleeping in the nest on the main floor, so I could easily hear his screams. The theme remained the same, only scarier each year. It was always a dream about an intruder who meant us harm. I was glad to know there were no weapons he could easily access as he fought off the bad guys without really waking up.

The spring of 2019 brought a new kind of storm to his brain. He began hallucinating in the daytime. The ones he had in the daylight were all benign. He might see the same fat doe grazing quietly on the fence line. In fact, he saw the non-existent deer most mornings. I believed it was easier on both of us if I were to climb into his pleasant hallucinations with him, rather than argue about reality. He would say, "Mag. Mag. Come here and look at this beautiful deer, see how shiny her coat is? I wonder if her fawn is nearby." I would agree with him and say, "Oh yes, she's a beauty. There must be plenty for her to eat and I bet her baby is just below the hill." He would smile and go back to whatever he was doing, and I didn't have to alert him to his failing brain. Win-Win. I often thought that if a loved one suddenly started having violent nightmares or sweet daytime visions, it would be difficult not to try to convince them of reality. Since Rockey's brain had dabbled in unreality for so long, by the time these hallucinations became almost a daily occurrence, I wasn't frightened by the change and felt no need to correct him. What good could have come from those corrections? It was simply part of the whole.

Rock never came back physically, either. He was less steady and never tried to walk without his cane or the walker. His stamina remained low long after he came home. He slept more often and for longer periods and some days just watched TV all day. Inches. He was going away by inches.

Journal Entry

Spring 2019

I was trying to talk myself down from an all too familiar ledge. Running the facts, the pictures, the looming future of my life against the imaginary life over the ledge. It occurred to me that no one would have designed this chapter of life as a goal.

As in, "When I get to be 60-something, I'd like my world to be full of waiting, watching, listening. I hope to find I've spent my life with someone who seems to have no respect for me or my well-being."

The life over the ledge is brimming with hikes in towering forests over cool, mountain creeks or seeing colorful desert dirt beneath my feet. Over the ledge I sway and stomp and dance to live music in small, intimate venues wearing cool shirts and my favorite boots. I eat eggs or crackers or just some ripe, sweet fruit for dinner. My sleep is uninterrupted, the dogs are allowed to bark sometimes, and I am mostly alone with only the dogs to care for. Over the ledge I am spontaneous and laugh more ... like before.

Before.

Before was busy and challenging, loving and laughing, frantic and rushing through life with arms wide open, trying to catch every experience. Before was vaguely fair; it had a rhythm and a balance to it. Work hard, make money, play hard. Sometimes, Before was even predictable and safe.

Some days I want to go over the ledge and make a life that resembles Before.

I went back to see the orthopedic surgeon after he had ordered a scan and one more X-ray of my leg in the last week of April, 2019. I sat in a chair in the small exam room and heard him knock, and I said, "Yeah?"

He opened the door and smiled big and said, "I see you've brought your bad attitude today."

I said, "Nah, I was just teasing, I'm always glad to see you."

He didn't mince any words and said, "The time is here. We agreed that if it didn't look better, you'd have another surgery. I think we should schedule it right away," he said, looking serious.

"Okay. Okay. When do you want to do this and what are you going to do to fix it?" I asked.

"I saved a spot for you on Tuesday and ..."

"Whoa!" I interrupted, "I can't be ready by Tuesday. I've got to find somebody to help us."

"Oh no, you won't need help this time. You'll walk out of here. This is a totally different deal than the first one," he said.

I squinched up my face and said, "Why is totally different?"

"No trauma this time. The trauma to your body when you came in last fall was huge. The impact of the fall, the surrounding tissue damage, the amount of time you laid on your side, you were in shock—we don't have any of that to deal with. You'll heal so much faster this time. That kind of trauma does wild things to healing. I swear, you'll be cooking dinner by Friday," he said, and he flashed one of his charming boy smiles.

I went in alone to check in for the surgery at 5:00 a.m. Tuesday morning.

He was right. The recovery was easy. I limped for a long time, but hours of PT and miles of walking built up strength and flexibility. Some muscles never quite returned, but others worked harder to make up the deficit. I have an asymmetrical butt because I lost so much muscle and a scar that runs from my right cheek almost to my knee, but was walking.

In August, Rockey set up the target for his bow practice before archery season. He was still a great shot and still wanted to look for elk. I was grateful, just like all the other years, that he still found joy in this season. He drove the Ranger to pick up his practice arrows. Fifty yards was too far to walk. He went up to his shack every evening from early September through Thanksgiving. I thought some habits are worth keeping.

My birthday, his birthday and Christmas all came and went with very little fanfare except for Andi and the Christmas evening. She laughed and tore off wrapping paper and hugged the old people and danced around in her Frozen jewelry. It was perfect.

And then it was 2020.

The Pandemic Arrives
2020

January of 2020 gifted us with mild weather and not much snow. I know it's not good for the environment, but it was a true boon to an aging farm couple. The gentle temperatures made all winter chores easier and trouble-free, everything from putting hay in for the horses and sheep to snow removal was possible with less wear and tear on the workers. Rockey still insisted on being the plow guy for the nine homes on our dead-end road. Each household paid him a small yearly fee to keep the road clear after every snowfall. I believe he continued this job because it was one thing on the ever-shortening list of things he could still accomplish. A winter with low snowfall and less wind, which can cause plow-bending snowdrifts, was great for his self-worth and didn't tax his body much.

I was continuing physical therapy and weekly sheep herding classes.

The year began easy. I had hopes of heading to Big Sky Resort just up the road and seeing if I still had any muscle memory for a few snowboard turns, but the blue-sky day with powder snow never materialized and my board hung unused in the garage. I wasn't interested in going unless conditions were perfect for a soft landing should I fall.

Everything changed when the coronavirus pandemic hit. I remember keeping several doctor and dentist appointments the week before everything began shutting down and feeling worried whether I should cancel all appointments. The information we all possessed would seem so inadequate months later, but I bought masks and began buying groceries through a delivery service. They didn't deliver way out here, but I was able to meet the delivery people at a friend's house. Was I supposed to wipe all these food packages down before I put them away? Should I wear gloves to handle this stuff?

It was the vagaries and conflicting reports on the coronavirus that shined a bright light on Rockey's dimming brain.

It's difficult to explain how I could live with him and be unsure about how deep his dementia ran, but there were many moments each day when he seemed quite normal. He had the same breakfast every morning, a small bowl of Honey Nut Chex or Cinnamon Life cereal. He drank the last of the milk from his cereal out of the bowl. He had a big cup of coffee with cream while checking the news and his email. There were lots of things he could do in a day that were the same things he had done when his brain worked perfectly, but COVID-19 was a conundrum for him. As the weeks turned to months, Rock would ask me at least once a week, "What's the name of the thing out there? I know it starts with a C." I would answer each time, "It's called COVID." Then he'd look puzzled and say, "Well, what is the other one, the one with the longer name?" I explained that "Coronavirus and COVID-19 are the same thing, just different names." He was quite worried about the virus and understood that he was considered High Risk, but he couldn't hang on to the facts about transmission.

Rock was surprised when I quit going to physical therapy and asked me why. I said, "Everyone there is a regular visitor of some clinic or hospital, and it seems to me that they are most likely to have contact with the virus. I think it's a germ festival and I'm not going back until we know more."

Even though he had been going to PT for over a year and had no improvement in his walking skills, he was reluctant to give it up. "They wipe everything down all the time. Doesn't that mean it's safe?"

I said, "It's probably safe until that guy who used to own the insulation company coughs or sneezes or even talks loud. He won't wear a mask and he's still out and about in restaurants and stores. They can't protect us from people who won't take the proper precautions."

A few weeks after I quit, one of the therapists tested positive and Rock quit PT too. After that, he started wearing his mask around the farm. In his truck, driving the tractor or the Ranger, there was Rockey in his own driveway, alone in a vehicle, wearing the plaid mask that my friend had made for him. He would stop by somewhere on the farm if I was working on something and he would be wearing his mask. As summer came on, the sun was bright and masks were hot, and I mentioned more than once that it was okay to not wear it on the farm. He would shake his head uncertainly and say, "I thought it lived in the air. Like it's everywhere, isn't it?" He waved his arm to indicate the sky all around us. I always tried again, "You can only get it from another person. From their breath and the droplets that come out of their mouth when they speak." He was never able to let go of his belief that it just floated around in the air, and you could get it if you were outside without a mask. As these conversations and questions were repeated over and over during the pandemic, I was quite surprised to be shown with such clarity what his brain could no longer process. It made me worry for his safety at a level I had not yet considered.

Nick had come by one summer evening and visited his dad in the shop. Rockey had gone back to the house and I was walking that way after chores when Nick stopped his truck to say hello. He mentioned Rock's weird mask wearing and I explained, "He just can't grasp that we get it from people. He thinks it floats around everywhere and he is very worried about getting it. I've been wondering if you've noticed any changes in him, besides the mask thing." Nick agreed that in his fragile condition, the virus would be devastating to Rockey and then we started to compare notes on small things he was having trouble with.

Nick said, "I had to hook up some hydraulic hoses for him on the bobcat. He kept trying to hook it up to the tractor and he kept missing the receiver."

I had a realization and asked, "Was his hand moving too wide to the right of the receiver?"

Nick thought for a minute and made a mock motion with his hand and said, "Yeah, he seemed like he couldn't see it and he was four inches to the right of where he should have been."

I took a big breath and said, "Oh wow. Something is going on in his brain. I've noticed the same kinds of movements, like he can't see what he's working on. But I just blew it off. What else have you seen?" We had a good talk comparing little changes we had both noticed but written off as incidental. Neither of us had any big ideas as to what might be causing these changes; there had been no singular health event, but we left with a gnawing feeling that something significant must be happening in Rockey's brain.

For the most part, we lived a solitary life on the farm long before COVID restrictions, so those changes toward isolation in the world didn't have a huge impact on us. We hadn't been to a restaurant in years, nor attended concerts together or gone to parties or social events. Other than the news reports becoming increasingly alarming, we remained unaffected until his granddaughter Andi's daycare had a positive COVID test from one of her teachers and closed for two weeks. We quit seeing Andi for her weekly visits because of the potential exposure, and Rockey seemed to drift away with that loss.

One night in August, we were sitting outdoors on the shady side of the house, and he said, "The babies. What about the babies?"

with a choking sob.

I looked over at him, surprised to see tears, and said, "What do you mean about the babies? Why are you so sad, Rock?"

He took in a ragged breath and said, "Do you think the babies will miss me?"

I began to rub my face like I do when I'm trying to control my emotions and I replied slowly and softly, "Why do they have to miss you? Do you mean because of COVID?"

He shook his head never meeting my eyes and said, "No, I mean when I'm dead. I have to kill myself soon now."

More face rubbing, and harder rubbing. I asked, "Why now?"

He said in a firmer voice, "Do you think they will miss me?"

I hesitated and said, "No, Rock. Andi is too young to understand the concept of death. She will miss you for a while, but she won't be able to grasp your death as being final until she is older. And Elliot is just too young to get it at all. I'm sorry, but that's just the way it is with kids. But they will know you through stories and photos and the memories their parents keep alive." I repeated my question, "Why now?"

He started crying in earnest and said, "Don't you see? My life is shit. I can hardly walk. I'm scared all the time. Half the time, I don't know what day it is, and I watch TV for hours a day because I can't do anything anymore. I told you back when I was diagnosed that I wouldn't live like this. Well, here I am, and I've stayed too long. This is no kind of life." I started to say something, and he looked me in the eyes through his tears and reminded me, "You promised me way back then that you wouldn't try to talk me out of it when the time came. I'm telling you, now is the time."

I looked at the ground, feeling stunned by his clarity, and watched my own tears fall to the concrete. I went to him and took him into my arms and didn't say another word. This wasn't even close to our first conversation about suicide, but it was the first time he said it was time for him to leave this world. I didn't ask how or when because it seemed too harsh, too coarse, even for me to say those words.

August was the time when Rockey set up his archery target by the driveway, carefully spraying lines on the ground with neon orange paint, the yardage marks to his target. He didn't walk back and forth anymore but used the Ranger. He would start at the thirty-yard mark, shoot three arrows and drive to the target to retrieve them, checking his accuracy. When he was satisfied with his proficiency, he would move farther back. I was walking up from the barn one day and he was just driving up to the target. He stood on wobbly legs, holding onto the Ranger for support, grinning wide and said, "Come here, check this out," pointing at the arrows in the target. There were two arrows touching together in the bullseye and the third was about an inch away from that sweet center spot.

I smiled up at him and said, "Wow, hotshot! How far away were you?"

He stood a little straighter, resembling that confident guy with the killer smile that I used to know, and said, "Sixty yards—can you believe it? I can barely tie my shoes, but I can still shoot an arrow and hit the target at sixty yards." I laughed and shook my head and stuck my hand up for a high five. He tried to meet that hand and missed, and we both fell into belly laughs at the irony, just for a minute.

Running Otters and Delilah

All through October, Rockey remained in that vague fog I found him in. His expression lost the look of fear, but he was far away in his mind. He went to his hunting shack every day during the archery season and continued into the gun season, but he suddenly stopped going out. When I asked him why, He only shrugged and said, "No elk."

The week before Thanksgiving, during the unusually warm fall, he headed up to the shack to resume his watch for elk. On the evening of November 20, he came back to house at sunset. I had dinner ready, and we ate like we always did, sitting in the big recliners, watching the news. Then he did something unusual, he tilted his chair back and fell asleep. Hard asleep. Rock napped some every day, but he never napped in the evening, thinking it would ruin his night's sleep. After a little more than an hour, I said, "Rock, wake up. Your show is coming on." No response, so I tried again, a little louder this time. Again, he didn't move. I got up and went to him and gently shook his shoulder. He blinked a couple times, powered his chair into the upright position and got up. He then abruptly turned, walked behind the chair toward an outside wall and walked into it.

I hurried to him and grabbed his arm to steer him and said, "Whoa wait, where are you going?"

Looking bewildered, he said, "I need to go to the bathroom."

Growing alarmed, I made my face calm and firmed up my grasp, leading him back around the chair and pointing us toward the bedroom. "Here you go. Did you just get up too fast?" I asked.

He mumbled, "Don't know. I feel really weird."

I let go of his arm to go through the doorway and he froze and started to tip over. My shoulder replacement wasn't even two weeks old and still had staples in it, so I grabbed him hard around his chest with my good arm and slammed him against the open door to keep him from falling. I didn't have a very good hold of him, and I said, "Okay. Gimme a second here." I repositioned myself, trying to guard my left arm, and said, "We're going to walk to the bed. Easy little steps." And I called them out with each step. "Step. Step. Step. Okay, stop and try to turn toward me, I will help you. Please don't grab this arm." And I held up my left hand. He took a firm hold of my right shoulder, turned clumsily around to face me and I told him he was safe to sit down. Sitting on the edge of the bed, I looked hard into his eyes to see if I could notice any changes. He only looked very surprised and after a moment or two I asked, "What happened just now?"

He shook his head in wonderment and said, "I just couldn't move my feet, so I tipped over, I guess. I feel so weird."

I said, "Okay, let's check some things." I started to do the simple neurological tests I had seen his doctors do dozens of times. I asked him to follow my finger as I moved it in front of his eyes, right to left. I asked him to make a smile. It was more like a grimace, but it was equal on both sides. I had him tap his thumb to each finger and it was easier for him on his right side, just as it had been for years. "Hold your arms out and touch your nose. Close your eyes and touch your nose. Raise your arms. Lower the right. Lower the left. Resist my pressure on your fists." I asked him to do all these things and found no glaring weakness on one side or the other. I asked him, "You feel weird how? Is your head buzzing or ringing? Do you feel dizzy or sick?"

He replied with a dazed look, "Yeah. All of those things a little, but I can't explain how weird I feel." We sat not talking for a few minutes and he said, "I still have to go to the bathroom."

I asked if he wanted help, and he said no, so I watched as he made his way, clutching the dresser, then the doorframe, then the counter.

He wanted to come back to the living room and sit in his chair, so I helped him get comfortable. We watched some TV, and the evening was uneventful. At about 9:00 p.m., he said, "I think I'll go to bed. I'm really tired."

I got his meds out for him, set his phone nearby and got some water for his nightstand, threw back the covers and tucked him in. He looked childlike in that moment, wide-eyed and worried. I stroked his worried face and asked, "Do you think you'll be okay in here?"

He nodded and said, "What do you think happened?"

I shook my head. "I don't know, Rock. Your sides are equal, but maybe a small stroke or one of those tiny seizures you used to have." I moved his phone and the TV remote and placed them on top of the comforter near his left hand. I showed him where they were and said, "Just call me if you get into trouble. I'll be downstairs, but I'll come right away." His eyes looked heavy and sleepy, and I kissed him gently and left.

I never heard any crashes or screaming in the night, and I lay awake for most of it.

In the morning, I didn't hear him thumping around, so I came up the stairs quietly. He was sitting up in bed pointing a remote at the TV and said, "My TV doesn't work again."

I took the remote and pushed a few buttons and the picture appeared. I looked around and saw that all the covers from the king-sized bed were on the floor in a giant twist. I said, "Oh my. What happened?"

"I got wrapped up like a cocoon and couldn't get out, so I just pushed it all onto the floor. Sorry," he said.

I started to pick the heavy mess up and said, "It's all right, I'll get it put back together. You want some coffee?"

"Yeah!" he said with a little smile.

I watched him closely when he moved to his chair as I fixed us some coffee. He seemed to be moving without any great difficulty, but he still had that funny, wide-eyed look on his face.

An hour or so later, I was in the kitchen peeling apples to make an apple crisp and he came in and leaned on the counter and watched for a minute, then said, "I'm going to kill myself today."

I looked up briefly and kept peeling, saying, "What's the rush? Why today?"

He very matter of factly said, "Whatever happened has turned my brain to mush and I think I should."

I countered with, "I can take you to the ER and they can take a look at you."

He snorted and said, "When has the ER ever been able to figure out what's going on with my messed-up brain? And isn't there that virus in the clinics and stuff?"

I had to agree that the ER didn't have a history of helping him with brain issues and yes, COVID exposure was a risk. I tried again, "How about if I call Echi on Monday and see if he can see you? You seem pretty normal; what does it feel like to you today?"

He closed his eyes and said, "I can't even say. I just know I am really fucked." Silence between us and I continued the apple preparation. Then he said, "Okay. I'd see Echi." Then he went back to the living room and watched TV. Not ten minutes later, he reappeared leaning on the counter and said, "I'm going to the garage and start the cars and gas myself."

I set my knife down and took a big breath and said, "I thought you were going to wait and try to get an appointment with Echi next week."

"No, I don't want to," he said.

I sighed and told him, "Well you can't tell me how and where you're going to do it and you sure can't do it in the attached garage. What kind of fool would I be to not notice cars running twelve feet from the kitchen? I'm pretty sure I'd be expected to call the sheriff if I knew you were trying to kill yourself in the garage. So, you have to quit telling me. Love you bad, honey, but I'm not going to prison for you." He seemed to accept that and returned to his chair.

Another couple of hours passed and I heard him in the laundry room just as he called my name. I walked in and he had shoes on and a jacket. I asked, "Where are you off to?"

He answered, "I'm going to the shop to see what's in there that I can start up and kill myself. But I'm having some trouble here. Can you fix it?"

I took a better look and saw that he had his jacket on backwards and his shoes on the wrong feet. I smiled and said, "Here, let me help you," and we got the jacket off and turned around. I said, "Your shoes are on the wrong feet. Do you care?"

He snorted and said, "I can't walk anyway, so I don't think it matters much."

I looked at his face, trying to keep my expressions neutral and said, "Remember I said you have to quit announcing your plans to me or I have to call the sheriff. Why don't you take off that coat, come back in and have some warm apple crisp and ice cream?"

He smiled like a little boy, and his eyes lit up and he said, "Oh. I love apple crisp."

I had foiled his plans one more time.

He napped for several hours, and as the sun dropped behind the mountains, I was grateful for nightfall. Later, I helped him into bed and covered him with a lighter version of covers and left the bottom untucked for easy escape, then gathered up my pillows and a blanket from my bedroom and took up residence on the couch. I thought I should stay close in case he had trouble. One full night of sleep felt luxurious when morning rolled around.

His confusion seemed to have deepened overnight, and he became obsessed with having to pee. He would announce where he was going and head for the master bath every fifteen minutes or so.

I asked him what was going on and he replied, "I just have to pee, but I can't go."

"Is it something that has happened before?"

He shook his head no. As the day went on, his focus on it became more singular. He would barely sit down, and he would get back up and head to the bathroom. At one point, he called my name, and I went to him, and he was standing in front of the toilet with his pants up, staring down, and he said, "I can't remember what I'm supposed to do."

I said, "Can you stand up to pee or do you want to sit down?"

He answered, "I'm so unsteady, I'm awful afraid I'm going to fall. Maybe I should sit down."

"Okay, good idea." I had him move aside and I showed him, step by step, how to grab the window frame and then the safety bar, take one backwards step and sit down.

He did all that and then said, "Now what?" and I thought my heart might break in two.

Not having any experience in this realm, I guessed and said, "Push your wiener down between your legs and pee. I'll leave you alone."

I still can't quite put a name on what I felt that day. I was so sad that something automatic had left his brain and now he had to think it through each time. I was scared, because if something this automatic was gone, what else had fallen out of his brain? As my own mind began to whirl with *What Ifs?* and *Now What Will We*

Do? questions, I quieted myself by asking what do I need to know in the next five minutes?

I knew that somewhere along the line, Rockey needed to use Depends. I was sure we still had a big package, and I looked through closets until I found them. My hope was that wearing these would dial back his anxiety a little. When he came out, I suggested that he wear one and then he wouldn't need to be so worried. He was glad for the idea, and I helped him change into sweats with some Depends underwear. He still hadn't been able to pee, and I said, "I have a remedy, come sit in your chair." I poured a big glass of water and squeezed a whole lemon into it and took it to him. He sniffed it and said, "What is it?" I told him it was just lemon juice in water and that it was a natural diuretic. Oh, disbeliever that he is, he had a look of suspicion. I laughed and said, "Girls know tricks like this. Just go with it. You'll see." Of course, it worked like a charm, and he was immensely pleased with his bathroom success.

It was Sunday, which was garbage gathering day at our place, so I started going room to room to get all the trash. This was another job he had been very attached to, and he stood and snatched a small bag out of my hand as I walked by and said, "I can do it." The big blue trash can was at the end of our half-mile driveway where the service picked it up it on Monday mornings. He would take the Ranger with the trash in its dump box and transfer it into the big blue can. Easy-peasy and he had done it every Sunday for years. I watched him drive away, pleased that he was steering straight, then went back to doing something else. I realized after twenty minutes or so that he hadn't come back, and I looked out the window to see if I could spot him. He was just pulling away from the shop and coming toward the house. I didn't want him to know I was watching him, so I got busy again. More time passed and he never came in the house. I looked out the window again and he was just sitting in the Ranger. I thought maybe he was talking on his phone, and I quit watching. Finally, I heard the door from the garage open and he sat down on the bench to take off his shoes. I called around the corner and asked, "How did that go?" I stepped closer and saw that familiar look of panic and fear in his eyes again.

He said, "The trash can was gone and then I got lost on the driveway."

I looked down our long driveway and could see the big blue can at the end of it. "Oh no," I said. "Where could it have gone? What did you do with the trash?"

He said, "Somebody must have stolen it. I put the trash in the shop can."

I said, "Good thinking," as I stood there looking at the trash bags in the back of the Ranger. I could feel my heart race a little and my chest getting tight as I wondered what the implications of his bat shittery crazy brain were going to be. Deep breaths, I told myself. What do I need to do right this minute? I helped him to his chair and no sooner was he seated before he was up and off to the bathroom again. I was nearly done preparing a favorite chicken and wild rice dish for dinner, threw together a salad and set the chicken in the oven to finish. He was walking back to his chair as I was putting on my coat, and I said, "Dinner will be ready soon. I'm going to run down and do chores before it gets dark. I'll be right back."

I took the trash to the big blue can, sitting right where it had been for over sixteen years, did my chores and went back to the house. Rockey managed to eat a child's portion of food, but said he liked it. He wasn't eating much these past few days. The evening was peaceful except for the obsessive bathroom trips. I counted seven trips in the first hour then tried to quit paying attention.

Monday morning, I called Dr. E's assistant and left a message about what was going on with Rockey's health. I had a sneaking feeling that he was going to be out of town, and I jokingly said on the message, "Somehow, I know you're going to call me back and tell me he's in Ethiopia again." When she returned the call, I could hear laughter in her voice as she said, "You know our good doctor pretty well. He is in Ethiopia providing neurological services again. But he will be in Bozeman on Tuesday, December 1ˢᵗ. We are totally booked, but I know he will make room to see Rockey. I will call you Monday with a time." I thanked her profusely and told Rock. He was dismayed that it was more than a week out, but Echi was the one doctor who knew his complicated medical history the best, so we agreed he was who Rock should see.

I'd like to say we settled into living with his now very scrambled brain, but there wasn't much settling about it. He brought up suicide every day. His sleep became disrupted and disturbed by increasingly violent and frightening night terrors. His bathroom obsession only got stronger with each passing day. I continued to sleep on the couch because I was afraid for his safety. He now had day hallucinations and they were soft and pleasant.

Every day around mid-morning, he would call out my name and say with some excitement, "Mag, come here. You have to see this." For several days, he saw a whitetail doe. I concurred that she was lovely. My favorite happened on a sunny Wednesday the day before Thanksgiving. He called to me, and I walked to his chair. He said, "I know this one is going to sound unbelievable, but I really think it's real."

"What is it?" I asked.

He motioned to me and pointed out the window at a place just past some pine trees. He was animated as he told me, "I saw three otters running down the field toward the canal. They were carrying a huge piece of poly and it was streaming out behind them as they ran. Do you see anything out there?"

I made a show of looking intently and said, "No, I don't see them, and I can't see any tracks. Was it the clear stuff, like construction poly?"

He said excitedly, "Yes, that's it exactly. I have a big roll of it in the shop, maybe they got it there."

I nodded sagely and said, "That's probably it. Were they running on all four legs or just on their hind feet?"

He loved this question and replied with his eyes lit up, "The two on the outside were running standing up on their back feet, holding the poly in their little hands. The one in the middle had the poly in his teeth. I think it was his job to keep it from dragging." His smile was fading, and he said, "Are you sure you don't see them? They looked so real."

I stared at his old-man boyish face and asked, "Would you like it if I went outside and looked to see if I can see them or the tracks?"

Happy again, he said, "Oh yeah. That would be great."

I pulled on some boots and walked through the snow out to the field, making sure I would appear in his line of sight. I came back into the house and said, "Sorry, dude. I didn't see them or find any tracks."

His sad smile cracked my heart a little and he said quietly, "Damn. They looked so real. It would have been cool if they had really been there."

I smiled and kissed his forehead and agreed that it would have been way cool. Moments like these were innocent ramblings and they felt sweet to me and not scary at all. I was comfortable not arguing with his hallucinations when they were benign. He seemed happy in them, and I saw no reason to dissuade him. Those happy sightings couldn't hurt a thing. When he landed in a terrifying hallucination, I used all my power to comfort and soothe him and words of reason to try to bring him back to safety. As the days went on, he started to see more frightening things than sweet wildlife imaginings.

One morning I went in to offer some coffee and he was sitting on the edge of the bed, looking at a pair of socks. He held them up and said, "What do I do with these?"

With no hesitation I smiled and took the socks from him and said, "How about I help you with these? It's a long way for you reach those feet."

"Socks," he said. "Nice." And he smiled like he remembered an old friend. I held out my hand to help him up and he was worried right away, asking, "Where is my cart? What happened to my cart?"

I steadied him as he stood and reached out and pulled his walker toward him. As he stood, my eyes got wide when I saw what he was wearing. He had on three pull-on Depends over a pair of cut-off sweatpants, over a pair of heavy cotton sweatpants and I assumed over some additional under things. I said, "Oh gosh, Rock. What do you have going on here?" He looked down and I could tell he wasn't quite sure, and I asked, "Is all that a little uncomfortable?" He nodded like a child, and I asked, "Would you like some help fixing it so it's not so bulky?" Again, the sweet childlike nod. I helped him take off his many layers of protection, I put less pants back on him and went to the living room to get him that cup of coffee I had promised.

I had ordered a turkey dinner for Thanksgiving from my friend Marci who prepares the best home-cooked meals anywhere. Marci delivered the boxes of goodness the day before, and I asked Rock if we should just start eating it now, and he said, "Why not? I don't even know what county I'm in, let alone when national holidays are." We feasted on turkey, stuffing, gravy, and mashed potatoes cooked every which way for days. I ordered an extra container of mashed potatoes, so I had plenty to make them my favorite way. Rockey could only eat small amounts for some reason, so we had tiny meals more times a day. We ate pumpkin and pecan pies with real whipped cream any time we wanted. There truly are foods that give comfort, and we took all the comfort we could get.

I stayed close to the house except for doing chores. Rock seemed so fragile, so weak and so confused I was always concerned that without supervision, he might fall or become frightened and do something that would cause him harm. A physical injury on top of his turbulent brain was too much to consider. I had just gotten the staples removed from my shoulder replacement the day he experienced what I called his Brain Explosion, until we found out for sure what had happened. The only caveat my surgeon gave me was, "Be very careful with it for four months, then you can do whatever you want." On Thanksgiving Day, I was only sixteen days out from that surgery, and it was hard to juggle my own best interests against Rockey's immediate needs. Not for the first time in our lives, showering Rock became a mildly dangerous excursion for both of us. It never got any easier for me to dance a man who was nearly a foot taller, with unreliable balance, into and out of a shower without somebody getting hurt. The near misses of him falling were adrenaline-producing events. I was still wearing a big sling on my arm and taking it off for the shower production left me feeling less safe from some sudden movement. I can smile about the silliness of it now, but on shower days, it produced some angst.

I became exhausted from the constant care he required and felt physically unable to keep up with his needs. The night terrors were happening every night now and I would wake and try to help him through them or out of them. He continued to have big trouble with the covers on his king-sized bed, getting tangled when he tried to get up. I cut a couple of blankets in two so there would be less bulk for him to deal with, but even that wasn't an adequate solution.

In one of his more lucid moments, he asked, "Are you going to put me in a nursing home? I know I am a total pain in the ass, but please don't do that."

I sat close to him and took his hand and said, "Yeah, you are a bit labor intensive, but we've talked about this before. I promised I would not do that to you."

He looked worried and said, for the first time ever, "But you can't keep doing this, can you?"

I said, "No. I can't, and I need help now. But we can't afford to pay for help with our regular household income."

"I have the money," he said.

"Well okay then. Order us some help," I replied.

He gave me a weak smile and said, "It's that money market account that you've been pissed off about forever. I was saving that for this situation so we could pay for home care."

"Great," I answered. "But my name isn't on it, and I can't use it."

"We can add your name, right?" he asked.

We were going to see his doctor the next day and I said, "Sure, we can go to the bank after your appointment."

He was relieved and said, "Find whatever you need. There is enough to pay for whatever help you need to make it easier for you." I agreed and started making phone calls right away.

I had not had good experiences with the national chains of home health care in the past, so I reached out to my friends looking for recommendations of people who might help or point me in the direction where I might find help. There is a difference between needing in-home medical care or in-home companion care. Rockey did not require medical-level care, but someone to hang out with him, make him something to eat and perhaps help with showering. Somehow in this flurry of phone calls and texts, I received a few pieces of gold. One was the name of a woman who had started her own home healthcare service. From her, I hired enough people to help Rockey for fifteen hours a week. From another place, I found Delilah. She had recently graduated from Montana State University with a degree in Civil Engineering. Because of COVID, Delilah had some time and a need for extra income. I got her name from someone I trusted greatly and called her right away. She came to us the next morning. She entered, in all her tiny-bodied fierceness and mask, greeted me, and I asked her to pull down her mask so Rock could see her face. She walked to him and said, "Hi Rockey, I'm Delilah and I'm here to help you guys. What can I do for you to make your day better?" Rockey smiled and said softly, "I'd like a grilled ham and cheese and some milk. Maybe some cookies."

And that was it ... she cooked that up and when I left, she was in a hard-backed chair with her legs pulled up underneath her, sitting very close to Rock to better hear his whispery voice. For someone who had never done home health care, this wonderful human possessed a most unusual gift.

There were a couple others who came and took good care of Rock while I ran errands or just drove to my favorite trailhead and walked with the dogs in winter silence. I knew his days were waning and I meant to do the best I could for him. These small breaks for a few hours were just the right mix of respite and fuel. I could walk back into the house feeling like I could take full breaths again.

I'll Die This Year
December 2020

By the time we got to the appointment with Dr. E, poor Rockey was edgy and even more confused than earlier in the day. I needed to get a wheelchair for him from the lobby and we didn't have to wait long. Full COVID protocols were in place, and I think that contributed to his confusion. He couldn't recognize people he'd known for years because of the face masks. When Echi came into the little room and dropped his mask for a moment, Rock visibly relaxed to see his favorite, trusted doctor. Echi noticed that Rockey's speech had changed dramatically since their last visit. The doctor always directed questions at both Rock and me and had made his intentions clear years ago. He told Rock that he could better assess his condition if he had input from me, because I saw different things and I wouldn't fib about them, so it wasn't odd or uncomfortable for me to me a part of the conversation.

"When did this voice change start?" he asked.

I answered, "It has been markedly growing quieter, I'd say, since last March."

"What happened in March?" he asked.

Rock pointed to his hip, and I said, "He had another hip re-placement in February."

He looked at each of us and said, "So how did that go?"

Rock rolled his eyes, and I said, "Exactly how I thought it would go for a guy with so many health compromises, Echi. He took nine days to come around from the anesthesia and to realize he was at home, and he has seemed slightly altered since then. The hip is no better and no worse even though he went twice a week to PT. He seems weaker and more disconnected to me. Sorry, Rock," I said, squeezing Rockey's hand. He made a weak smile and shrugged.

Echi looked at Rock and asked, "Do you agree?"

Rockey nodded sadly and said, "Yeah. Really weak and mixed up."

Echi sat down in front of Rock and said, "Okay. We're going to do some tests."

I laughed and bumped Rock, saying, "He probably has a bag of tricks we didn't know about when we tried."

Echi smiled and said, "Did you do this one, and this one?" He asked after each of the same ones I had done at home. I nodded. "What did you find?" he asked.

I said, "He seemed pretty equal on both sides. I didn't see any huge deficit in either side."

He smiled and said, "Now here come the tricks." He asked Rock to do some specific movements with the lower half of his legs and feet, and it was immediately apparent that one side couldn't do the tasks at all. After a few more tricks, he leaned forward and said in his deep voice and rich Basque accent, "Rockne, you've had a stroke." Rockey's face crumbled as tears began to fall and Echi looked at me and said, "Likely, the right side of his brain, affecting the left side of his body."

Choking a little, Rock whispered softly, "Can you fix it?"

Echi patted Rockey's knees and said, "No, Rockne, there is nothing to be done."

I asked, "Big or small?"

Echi replied, "There's no way to tell without a scan. Do you want a scan?"

"Rock?" He nodded and I said, "Yes, we want a scan."

He left the room and Rockey broke down in wracking sobs. I crawled into his lap and cradled his head and just held him. He said, "My dad."

"I know. But you are not your dad. The only difference between yesterday and today is that now it has a name and that doesn't change anything, Rock."

Echi came back and joked, asking, "You two kids want the room?"

Rock tried to wipe away his tears as I hopped down and said, "He's just having a rough time, Doc."

"Why, Rockne?" he asked, looking into Rock's eyes.

Rock stumbled as he tried to tell Echi, "My dad died of a stroke when he was sixty-eight. I'll be sixty-eight next week. I will die this year."

"Oh no, this one hasn't killed you, Rockne. Maybe stirred up your brain a little, but you're sitting right here." He handed me a piece of paper and said, "Do you know where this is? He can have a scan there in thirty minutes."

I said "Yeah, I know where it is, it's just fifteen minutes over that way. Then what?"

He said, "We will call you on our way back to Billings and I'll give you the results. Or Carrie will." Carrie was his capable assistant. "Okay, Rockne?" he said. Rockey nodded and I helped him into the wheelchair.

I drove over to Hell on Earth, aka Bozeman Health, to get him to the scan. The lot was full and a paper delivery truck was parked in the patient unloading zone. I drove around twice and finally double-parked, blocking the paper truck, and went in and got a

wheelchair for Rock. I set the chair by the curb and went to retrieve Rock and helped him to the curb. Just then, an old woman,
a woman my age, swooped in and snatched the wheelchair just beyond my grasp. I immediately sped up, half-dragging Rockey and
yelling at the woman to bring it back. Well of course she didn't,
leaving both of us sputtering obscenities as Rock hobbled toward
the door. I found a ledge for him to rest against and I went in
search of another wheelchair. He managed a laugh when I came
back pushing a brown, jumbo wheelchair. It seemed to be about
three feet wide and put together in the 1960s.

"What the fuck?" he mumbled as he slid into the rickety ride.

"Whatever is hardest for the patient, dear. That's our motto." We
both cackled a mean laugh.

He got out of the imaging lab and we headed for the bank. I had
called ahead, knowing the lobby was locked for COVID protocol,
so I parked and knocked on the glass doors. Two of the head bank
ladies opened the door and I said, "You'll need to come to my truck
for the signatures. Rock can't make it in here." They gathered the
papers and came outside, and Rock rolled down his window. He
signed some papers, I signed some papers and both ladies reached
in and touched him and said, "Be well, Rockey," and both started
to cry as they walked back inside.

We drove off and Rock dryly said, "Wow. I must look pretty bad
to make them cry."

I laughed and said, "Oh no. You know, the ladies all love to touch
the big Rock. You've been admired by them near and far for your
whole life."

We were both laughing hard now, and he whispered, "Yeah,
that's me. A real chick magnet. And I'm all yours, baby." We still
managed to laugh at the damnedest times.

Carrie, Dr. E's assistant, called as we were headed home. The
scan showed a stroke on the right side of the brain in the blah-
blah region, and the blah was also affected. I asked her to have the
radiologist mail me a copy of the report in layman's terms, please.

I believed the words I had said to Rockey. In this circumstance, knowing the name of it didn't really matter anymore. It was a permanent change.

Rockey wanted to lie down as soon as we got home, and I was grateful for a little quiet slice of the day. I googled what I thought Carrie had told me but was so far off, I might just as well have searched for blah-blah. I knew in my heart that Rockey's health status today would likely be the best he would be from here on out. His weight was dropping, he was less cognizant, he had less hours in every day where he could follow a conversation and less yet where he would contribute to one. He had not experienced incontinence, but his odd and obsessive behavior with peeing was getting worse every day. He decided he needed to change clothes each time he attempted to pee. I didn't try very hard to dissuade him. It seemed important to him, and it was harmless other than annoying me a little. He had not been able to dress himself at all since the stroke—shirts on backwards, both legs in one leg of pants, both arms in the neck of a shirt—so there was an ever-changing and always growing pile of clothes strewn about his bed if I didn't keep an eye on it.

That night after dinner, he handed me his phone and said, "Text people and tell them."

I took the phone and looked at him and asked, "Who do you want me to text and what should I tell them?"

He looked solemn and said, "You know who. The ones who need to know."

I opened his text app and started typing in names: Tim, Wally, Jeff, Bob, Tim, Rock, Olga, Dave, Susie and Ron, Roxann, Dave Johnson and not many more. I typed some text and we landed on something like this: "Hey everyone, this is Mag using Rockey's phone. Rock had a stroke on 11/20. He is home and kind of mixed up but doing okay. He doesn't want to talk to anyone because it's too hard for him to speak. You can call me or text back here and I'll answer any questions."

I only heard back from a few of them. One of things I find hard to forgive is how so many of the people who had been Rockey's friends when he was strong and healthy and funny and energetic withheld their friendship when his body failed him. I understand that, in our culture, we like to look away from disability. It is such a cheat to the person being disabled. I saw the same thing happen with my beautiful, eccentric and always entertaining mother. She had MS, and as that disease stole her mobility, her energy and her ability to speak clearly, the people who had been her friends slowly stopped seeing her. It broke my young heart for her, and it pissed off my old heart for Rockey. However difficult it may be to see people we care about diminished, imagine what it feels like to be that person.

Wednesday was quiet and ordinary. Rockey was still quite tired from the medical adventures of the previous day. Delilah came for a few hours and sat close to Rock and whispered with him again and fixed him something good to eat. Thursday was a new young woman named Angela, who had been doing home health for a decade. She had agreed to help Rockey shower and stayed with him for part of the day.

When I came home and she left, I asked Rock, "How did that go?"

He made a face, and I laughed and said, "What? Did she pinch you or hit you?"

He smirked and said, "No. The water was too hot in the shower, and I told her twice, but she didn't fix it. Then she just sat on the couch and stared at me."

I snorted with laughter at his indignance and said, "We never have to have anyone come here if you don't like them, you know."

He grinned a tiny grin and said, "Oh, she was okay. She's no Delilah. That's for sure."

I said, "I think we're both lucky to have found the one and only Delilah."

"Can't come every day?" he asked. I told him she worked another job and could only come a few times a week. He quietly said, "Damn. She's really cool."

"I know, and she'll be back before you know it."

When I helped him into bed that night, he was quiet and serious. He asked if I would sit with him for a while and I said sure. He asked me to give him a really good hug, and I did. I snuggled into his side and held him for a long time.

I asked him, "Are you scared?"

He said, "No. Just sad."

I stroked his chest and said, "You can be sad. You have every right to be sad." I laid there by him for a while until I felt him start to relax, then I pushed myself up and asked, "You okay if I go to bed now? I think I'll go sleep downstairs in my good bed for a change, if you think you'll be all right." I had moved permanently to my own room downstairs after my broken leg healed. I sometimes slept there for weeks at a time but would still sleep on the couch upstairs if I thought Rockey was bound to have trouble in the night. My room was on the opposite end of the house from Rockey's room and unless there was an enormous crash, I would never hear him. In these days of Rock's mind fading away, Zada had become a reliable alarm for me. If he started to move around in the night, she would thump her head on my arm until I woke up and went upstairs to investigate.

He said, "I'm tired. I think I'll sleep good tonight. You go get a good night's sleep too. Thanks for taking care of me." I kissed him goodnight and went down to my room.

Friday

I came upstairs about 8:00 a.m. and went to the kitchen to get some coffee. I got that going and went to Rockey's room to see if he was awake. I knew right away something wasn't right. He had a shirt on and was lying face down in his pillow. I knew he wasn't wearing a shirt when I left him the night before and he never laid on his stomach. I walked to him and could hear him breathing loudly into his pillow so I shook him. No response. I threw back the covers so I could roll him over and I saw pill bottles and pills and pill bottle covers under him and scattered on the sheet. It was impossible for me to roll him with only one good arm, so I pulled the pillow away from his face and tried to straighten his neck a little so he might breathe better. I called 911 and told them that my husband had tried to kill himself and they should send an ambulance. The dispatcher asked me some questions and told me to roll him over. That took a little while and when I got back on the phone, she asked me if I could do compressions. I told her no because I had just had a shoulder replacement and unless I could do compressions with one hand, I couldn't do it. She asked what he had taken and where he got the pills. I recited the drug names from the bottles and picked up the old zip lock bag they had all been in. I said, "He must have gotten the bag of leftover prescriptions for pain from old surgeries. There were a few oxys, some hydrocodone, some Flexeril, but I don't think any of these had very many pills in them." She asked where they had been kept and I answered, "In a cupboard in the bathroom, where they have been for years."

Pretty soon, the EMTs started coming up the driveway and into the house. My experience with these people had always been good, but the atmosphere was different this time. Nobody looked at me or asked any questions. Some dude with a clipboard was walking around picking up this and that, and I said, "Excuse me, who are you? Are you with them?" He shook his head. I said again, "Excuse me, but you're in my house and you're not working on my husband, so who are you? My name is Maggie and that guy in there is my husband Rockey and you need to stop touching stuff until you tell me who you are."

He still didn't look at me but said, "I'm busy, ma'am," as he scribbled on his clipboard. I told him he was rude and presumptuous to be in my house without any apparent job and without properly identifying himself.

Good neighbor Bob had followed them up the driveway, and he stood beside me in my living room and said, "Mag. It's okay."

I leaned in and said, "It's not fucking okay, Bob, but I'll back off."

I heard the EMTs say his vitals were strong, heartbeat and respiration were good. Somebody asked whether Rock had a health directive, and I answered yes. They asked me to find it. I rolled my eyes secretly and wondered where the hell that piece of paper might be. They loaded him onto the gurney, and Zada tried to get in the ambulance with him. I don't know who all was there, but I saw for the first time lots of cars and trucks with lights on them in my driveway. I called Zada out of the ambulance and they closed the doors. I think it was a sheriff's deputy who asked if I wanted to ride with him. I said no that I needed to find the health directive and put some real clothes on and that I would follow. I went back in and tore through a file drawer and found a big binder from the attorneys. I flipped through the huge document and found the page, tore it out and made a couple copies. I folded them and stuck them in my jeans pocket. I hurried to the bedroom and looked at the mess and turned around, put the dogs in my truck and left to follow the caravan leaving our place. I don't remember seeing Bob again.

By the time I got into the ER and found Rockey, a doctor was hooking him up to something, and I said, "No. No. You can't do that." I took the paper out my pocket and said, "It says so right here."

The doctor looked at the official health directive that was notarized and had a case number registered to the State of Montana, tossed it aside and looked scathingly at me and said, "That doesn't mean anything now. I can void it in the case of suicide."

I raised my voice and said, "What do you mean? This is supposed to be an official document. What good is it to have one if you can just ignore it?" He abruptly dropped everything and stormed from the room. I quickly dialed Steve, a long-time friend and attorney in Minneapolis whose firm had drafted Rock's will and this health directive. He said to put him on the phone with the doctor, which I did when the asshole came back into the room. He still wouldn't look me in the eye.

Something changed, I can't quite remember what. Steve's call was back in my ear and Steve said, "Mag, the doctor told me you were upset that he was trying to treat Rockey. You need to stop yelling at him."

The doctor left the room again and I whispered angrily at Steve, "What the fuck, Steve? Stop yelling? What is this guy, a five-year-old? He's trying to violate Rockey's health directive, which specifically states no life saving measures be taken and he's worried about me yelling?"

Steve quietly responded, "Mag. Call me when you get out of there." And hung up.

The doctor came back and said they would be taking him to a room. I asked how Rockey was doing. He said his heartbeat was strong and breathing was good. I asked how long until he would be in a room and where it would be. He ignored me, and I said, "I'll be back."

I started down the hall and was stopped by a sheriffs' deputy, who said, "The detectives want to talk to you. Suicide, you know."

I didn't know, but I looked around and said, "Okay. Where are they?"

He said, "Oh no, ma'am, they're not here. You'll have to come down to the station. You can ride with me."

I said, "No thanks. I'll drive. I've got the dogs in my truck. Where is the station?"

He told me and told me to follow him, so I got in my truck, nearly ready to throw up. I dialed Steve and told him where I was headed and that I was plenty freaked out. His advice was, "Be careful what you say and don't lose your temper, Mag." I said something like, "Sure, Steve, and everyone in the medical world has treated Rockey like a prince. I'm mad just being in the parking lot of a hospital, Steve. The chances are low that I won't lose my temper because I'm already furious. What new hell is this, being questioned by detectives?"

Steve said, "The doctor thought your behavior was odd, and he told the deputy that he thought you tried to kill your husband. I'm not a criminal lawyer, Mag, but I'll find you one."

Shaking now, I said to Steve, "I didn't have anything to do with this. This is just nuts."

"Watch what you say and don't get mad. Call me when you are done."

Now I was really freaked out. I followed the deputy car to the Law and Justice Center and realized I had been here once to pay a speeding ticket. I was glad that masks were required just so I didn't feel so obviously criminal. He took me to a room that could have been part of a television cop show set. It was a small gray cinder-block square with a rickety little table and two chairs and another chair in the corner. The observation window/mirror had a fist-sized smash in it with cracks radiating from the center. At least it didn't stink. I tried to sit still and not look at my phone. I felt like I waited at least a half hour for the detectives.

They introduced themselves, and I tried not to be weird. Since I may be a little sketchy on what constitutes "weird" in this situation, I can't imagine how I came off. I didn't cry here or at the hospital. Maybe that was weird. I suppose some would think so. They asked about Rockey, I told them briefly about the recent stroke and that he had Parkinson's. They asked if he had daily meds and I said, "Yes." They asked if I dispensed his daily meds and I said, "Yes." There were more questions and some repetition of questions. The guy sitting closest to me wasn't wearing a mask. I didn't dare say anything, but I tried to push my chair away from his face. More questions and always the one about the daily meds. I finally said, "What's going on here? What are you guys looking for?"

One of them said, "We're trying to decide if you were an accessory."

That was it. Weird or not, I stood up and said, "An accessory to what? A botched suicide and then I called 911 to save him?"

The masked one said, "Well you told us you dispensed all of his meds. How did he get those bottles open if you had to give him all his daily meds?"

Starting to get angry and trying not to raise my voice, I said, "I gave him his daily meds because he couldn't remember what he'd taken. And you never met Rockey Goertz. If you think a stroke would have kept him from opening a plastic bottle, you are way off base. He would have smashed them with his shaky old hands if he wanted to get them open. He didn't need me to open a bottle. I've had enough of this. Am I allowed to leave?"

They sputtered a little and said, "Yes, you can leave. We were just asking questions. But we'd like to come out to your house and the scene."

I said, "The scene is his bed, and I don't think I want you to come to my house. So, no. I should be at the hospital so I can be with my alive husband."

I turned and walked out, trying to look like a person who wasn't terrified might look. My hands and legs were trembling badly. As soon as I was out of the parking lot, I called good neighbor Bob and said, "Bob, I really fucked up. You have to tell me what to do." Bob was a retired Federal Marshall, so I figured he'd know cop stuff. I told him the detective story and what I said when I walked out.

Bob said, "Mag, you need to call that detective back and tell him you were under great duress, and he can come out, right now, if he wants to. And you know, some tears might help."

I rolled my eyes at the stupid drama I was expected to perform, knowing that it probably would help. Yuck. "Geez, Bob. I was under duress. Why do I have to apologize and why should I let them come to the house?"

He said, "Did you get mad, Mag?"

I wondered to myself why everyone kept asking me if I got mad. *I'll need to do a little self-reflection, I think, when this is over.* "I was a little mad, but I didn't swear, and I didn't yell. Fuck, Bob. I didn't help Rockey try to kill himself."

Trying to soothe me, Bob said, "I know you didn't. And they'll know it too. But if you don't let them come out now, they can get a search warrant and tear your house apart."

I am in a goddamn television cop show, I thought to myself. I took a big breath and said, "I got it, Bob. Thanks, I'll do my best. I'm calling you for bail." I started rifling through my pockets for the detective's card and swearing just a little about what Rockey had done and what position it had put me in.

I called the detective before I had even reached my driveway. I offered the duress excuse and even managed a snuffle or two. A wonderful friend named Laurie called just after I had my slice of humble pie with the detective on the phone. She swore a color-ful streak and said, "I can't fucking believe that we as women are expected to act like that and even more disappointing is that we know how to do it so well."

"Humph," I grunted. "You ought to be in my shoes. It feels cheap and whorey right now."

"Oh no," she said. "You don't get to feel bad by saving yourself with some required command performance. Survival, baby. If play-ing the lesser is what it takes to get you out of this, use everything you got, my friend. Fuck them. Fuck this misogynistic world."

"I love you, Laurie. Thanks for the grit. I gotta get ready and get my helpless persona out of the closet before they arrive. It won't do for me to be stoking my feminist pissed-off person. Later."

The detectives drove up the driveway just after I ended a call from Nick. He was so pissed, he wanted to come over and be there when the detectives were detecting. I said, "No, Nick. Stay away, or you'll get us both thrown in jail. I'll call when they leave."

I walked them to the bedroom and swept my hand to invite them in. It was the first time I had really looked at it, and I re-marked, "Wow. The EMTs don't clean up after themselves, do they?" There were discarded wrappers, bits of plastic somethings, a rubber tourniquet, a bloody syringe and other hazardous waste, all scattered about.

The detectives were touching things, looking at the bottom sheet with bits of pills and one of them said, "No. They usually leave quite a mess."

One picked up a bottle I had set on the dresser and read the label. He said, "Oh, this is from 2014."

I said, "Yeah, I told you it was a bag of leftover prescriptions for pain meds from knee surgery, a dental procedure, hand surgery. I bet you both have a stash of the same thing in your house. Every-body keeps them just in case you get hurt."

They seemed to have had enough detecting and said, "Okay, thanks for letting us in." As they walked out, they stopped to look at photographs in a bookshelf. There was Rockey skiing, then coming down the Big Couloir at Big Sky on a snowboard, both of us on a pack trip leading a string of mules, Rockey finishing concrete, one of us scuba diving and a beautiful photo of us together all dressed up looking like movie stars.

I said, "So are you guys going to arrest me now?"

They even looked a bit sheepish and said, "No ma'am."

I stiffened up and my anger resurfaced, and I said, "Good. Take a long look at those photos. I have loved that man since you two were in junior high. I've taken care of him every day for the past ten years. You asked me in that room, why on earth would he want to kill himself? Look at who he was. He can hardly walk to the refrigerator to put ice in his water cup now. He can't pee and he doesn't know what day it is. How dare you ask me why he would want to leave this world."

I opened the door for them to leave. Just then Nick pulled up, and I walked to his truck as the detectives stared while opening their car doors. I whispered to Nick, "Okay, you better hug me hard like I'm the best step-mom in whole world." He did and then we went inside.

Nick was awful mad that I had been accused, and he snorted, saying, "Well they sure didn't know anything about my dad. He would have used a claw hammer on his head if he couldn't figure out a better way." He asked what condition Rock was in and whether he should go see him.

"I don't know because I wasn't able to go back to see him after I was swept up in this clown show. At the very least, he will sleep until tomorrow."

Nick looked sad and said, "He'll be really pissed that it didn't work."

I agreed and said, "If he's ever conscious again. He might be gorked out forever. I'm not sure who they're letting in, COVID restrictions. It's your call. I expect to hear from somebody there. I'll go in right away if he wakes up."

Nick said if I thought it would help, he'd be happy to go see him. He hugged me and had a few tears as he drove away. It was getting close to 4:00 p.m. now and this day had left me with the ache of too much adrenaline. I felt a crash coming. I stripped the bed and threw every piece of bedding into the laundry room, starting a load of sheets. I opened every window in the bedroom on that December day and set up two fans on high speed and pulled the door closed. I felt the need to get rid of the tainted air. Tainted by the judging looks of the EMTs and the careless way they dropped refuse, by the sheriff's deputy staring at me, by the detectives touching Rockey's things. After I vacuumed and wiped off his nightstand, I kept the door closed, the windows open and the fans running all night. It felt like the right thing to do. I would smudge it more than once in the days to come.

A doctor called and said Rock was still unconscious, but his breathing and heartrate were strong and in the normal range. I asked if I should come. She said, "He's really out of it, and he won't know you're here. Take a break if you need to." Pause. "I understand you were put through the wringer today and I want to say how sorry I am."

I had been cold to her, but I softened and said, "Yup. Quite a coup for law enforcement to snag an old woman for unsuccessfully being an accessory to suicide. It doesn't even make sense when I say it out loud."

She stammered a little and then said, "The ER doctor who was working on your husband—the one who told the detectives he thought you acted suspiciously—he's a partner with me in our ER practice." I was silent. She went on, "I want you to know what he did was completely unacceptable, and I will be bringing it to the attention of our other partners."

I replied in a hard voice again, "Good. He was an arrogant prick totally ignorant of this slice of life. You guys should do some continuing ed on progressive, degenerative diseases and what that does to a person over a lifetime. That doctor was in over his head and way out of line. But thanks. I didn't even expect an acknowledgement of it, to tell you the truth." She seemed genuine and I was moved by the courage it took for her to break rank with the apology. She said she was on duty all weekend and would call me in the morning with an update. I thanked her and hung up with a sigh of relief.

Saturday, Rock never regained consciousness. I couldn't gather the courage to go visit, because I imagined a deputy coming out of a hallway to slap handcuffs on me. I talked to the hospital staff every couple of hours and told them I would come right away if Rockey awoke.

The doctor called early Sunday morning and said Rock was awake, but not making any sense. I asked, "Is he talking?"

She said he was, but they couldn't understand him. She told me, "He's having difficulty swallowing. I assume that's from the stroke."

"No. He could swallow just fine Thursday night. We had dinner and he was not having swallowing issues. It has to be from the narcotics."

"What do you want us to do? We've been afraid to give him anything more than juice because of the choking and he's now listed as DNR."

I said, "Well, maybe the swallow reflex got sedated in the effects of the drugs. I think you should give him some soft food. I believe he can recover his ability to swallow if we give him a chance. Tell whoever is with him to smack him hard on his back between his shoulder blades if he chokes. He's been choking for years. I'll shower and head that way right now."

She asked, kind of timidly, "Would you let me speak to you when you get here?"

I said, "Of course. I'll have someone page you."

I masked up, had my temperature checked and was escorted down some ghostly empty hospital halls to a ghostly empty ward with no personnel in sight. I crept along, quietly peering into doorways until I found Rock, sitting up in bed with his eyes closed. I said hello to the young woman sitting with him and walked to his side. His eyes remained shut tight and his lips were moving. I picked up his hand and stroked it and said softly, "Rock, it's me. I'm here." No acknowledgement came. I bent down to hear the whispers. I barked a little laugh and said, "Oh no you don't. You don't get to shave a year off your age, just because you're in the hospital, Rock. It's '52. You were born in '52."

I looked over at the girl, and she asked, "What was he saying? He's been saying the same thing for hours."

"He is saying 12/12/53, but his birthday is 12/12/52. You know, they ask patients that question twenty times a day. He's showing that he knows his birthday. Even though he had the year wrong. He is also pretending to be a much younger man." I squeezed his hand and he growled out, "HA!" and kept up his corrected birth-date whispery chant with his eyes closed tightly. I felt my heart constrict, and I walked to the window so he couldn't feel me crying or so a tear wouldn't fall on his arm, and he would have another chance to feel bad about what he was putting me through. He was probably still perceptive enough to know that, and I didn't want to clutter his broken mind with concern for me. I talked to him from the window with silent tears coursing down my face. I said, "You've got a helluva view here, Rock. You might want to open your eyes." He looked haggard and old and very skinny, and his lips just kept moving. I kissed him on the forehead and said I was going to leave. As I walked out the door, I looked up the hallway and saw a tall person wearing blue scrubs and a mask, running full tilt toward me.

As this person got closer, I realized it was a woman, and she stopped abruptly in front of me and asked, "Are you Maggie?"

I looked up into blue, blue eyes and said, "I am."

"I was afraid I would miss you. I am doctor so-and-so. I'm so glad to meet you. Can we talk for a minute?" I nodded and leaned back against the wall in the hallway. She repeated her confession about her partner's inappropriate actions, and her apology felt sincere to me. I accepted that apology. She asked, "Has anyone talked to you about end of life?"

I teared up immediately and said, "No. Not one person has ever spoken to me about the inevitable. I would be grateful for that conversation." I slid to the floor. She did the same across the hall. With our masks on and socially distanced, she and I began one of the most important medical conversations of this long, treacherous road I had traveled with Rockey.

She said, "Rockey's condition is unrecoverable. He may wake up or he may never be conscious again. His body will begin the dying process. It will begin to refuse food and then refuse water. The body knows its way to the end, and all we can do is try to keep him comfortable. I will register you with hospice and I'll notify you in an email. You must choose the hospice service you want. There are several in town and I suggest you talk to some friends who might offer any insights of the different agencies. If you have time to do that, I will set that up today. My goal would be to get Rockey home tomorrow. He will have to be transported by ambulance because he is too weak to get into a car. Hospice will come to your house tomorrow and help you get set up."

I said, "What about the necessary equipment? How do I get a hospital bed?" She asked whether I wanted him in a bedroom, and I said, "The living room is wide open, and we could access his bed from both sides there. And if he did wake up, he could look at our incredible views."

"Nice," she said. "Hospice will ask you what you think you need, and they will make suggestions. They will order it and have it delivered and set up before the ambulance arrives. A hospice coordinator will come to your home by the end of the day and talk with you about their services and what to expect."

I was uncharacteristically speechless.

She went on, "He may live a week or a month, but it won't be long. They will be with you every step of the way and help you navigate through this."

I stood and said, "Thank you for your candor. It's often in short supply with someone with as many broken parts as Rockey." She asked if she could hug me and I said, please do. I was enveloped in the best hug I had felt in ages and kind of wanted to just stay there feeling safe. I broke away and with teary eyes and thanked her again. I slipped into the room and whispered to Rock that he'd be home tomorrow and not to give anybody a hard time. He just kept his eyes closed and continued his birthdate chant.

It was a strange feeling I had driving away from the hospital that day. For once, I had no reason to hurry. I slowly drove the twisty backroads to my end of the Gallatin Canyon, trying to take notice of the beautiful place we called home. I had a picture in my head of the ambulance coming up our long driveway, bringing Rockey home for what would be the last time. I let that thought sit there in my head for a while and contemplated what the next few weeks might bring.

Delilah was scheduled to come to help Rockey in the morning. I texted her, told her there had been some changes and asked her to call me. When she did, I told her what had transpired and said, "This isn't what you signed up for and he isn't the same guy you took care of last week. I just wanted to give you the chance to back out if you want. It isn't going to be pretty." That brave young woman paused long enough to take a breath and said, "Nope. I'll see you at 9:00 a.m. I'm in this with you and Rock."

In the end, the ambulance wasn't scheduled to come until 2:00 p.m., so Delilah came later. The medical equipment company was good at communicating and showed up ahead of 2:00 p.m. with the hospital bed and various other helpful things. The ambulance service was less so. They drove up at about 2:45 p.m., and two baby boys hopped out. They opened the back doors and looked at me and said, "Can he walk?"

I probably made a stink face when I said, "No he can't walk. That's why you're driving him."

They grabbed ahold of the gurney and kind of slammed him to the ground and again, looked at me and said, "Can you help us?"

I snorted and said, "No fellas, I can't help you. You were hired by the hospital to bring this man home. Home means into the house … carried by you two wearing the ambulance uniforms."

Their innocent faces began to show the dawning of the realization that they were clueless as to how to accomplish this. They followed me into the garage pushing the gurney and looked at the three steps into the house as if it were Mt. Everest. "How do we do this?" one asked.

I told them that in the past, the lead guy folds up the wheels and legs and the bottom guy lifts his end up thereby keeping the patient level. They didn't know how to fold the legs up, so they just lifted and jostled and nearly dumped their cargo until they got both sets of wheels safely onto the laundry room floor. I looked back at Delilah, who was watching from the hallway, and gave her the Big Eyes as if to say, "Welcome to the circus." They wheeled Rock down the hallway, and then I had to coach them through the transfer from the gurney to the bed. It was one of the most ungainly and scary things I've seen. They jostled and juggled, Rock moaned with pain, they nearly dropped him on his head, but finally landed him on the bed.

Delilah stepped into the fray and said, "First day, guys?"

She was young and cute, and they blushed bright red and said, "Yeah."

"I thought maybe," she said as she turned to start trying to help Rock get comfortable.

I walked out with the baby boys and said, "Hey guys, I'm going to give you a little advice. Don't ever leave the hospital without knowing the condition of the patient you're carrying and information about the place you're taking them. They owe you that information. The hospital knew we had three steps. They should have told you. By the way, you might want to practice how to move the gurney around before you load up the next one. You were lucky today that he didn't fall right off."

They did a little toe scuffing and said, "Yeah, sorry about that."

I told them, "I'm not mad at you guys. Your bosses sent you off without the proper preparation. Don't let them put you in that position again. Someone will get hurt and they'll blame you two. Get what you need to do the job right. Okay?" I smiled at them, and they looked relieved.

Back inside, while Delilah was trying to tilt Rockey's head up and prop a pillow underneath it, I hurried and lifted his head and shoulders so she could place it. We fiddled around with raising and lowering his bed until we found what looked comfortable. We wrestled him into clean sweatpants and a shirt and slipped a pillow under his knees. Then we wheeled the bed around, so Rockey was facing a wall of windows looking over the broad expanse of the ranch next door.

Delilah put her head close to Rockey's and asked, "Rock, do you want some ice water?"

"Yes, please," he said in his breathy voice.

She looked at me and smiled, saying, "Coming right up."

I left those two alone for a little and stepped outside to gather myself. I wasn't able to rid myself of an uneasy feeling of what was coming. This might be a much bigger job than I had imagined.

The hospice lady, Jan, came shortly after. She was only there briefly to assess us, but she left me with a teaspoon of confidence that I would have someone to ask, someone to deliver the care he would need to get through this. I asked her when the helpers would arrive. She looked surprised and said, "Oh honey, we don't have helpers. You have to hire them on your own. Janelle will come every other day to help keep Rockey clean and comfortable. We give you the medications he needs to be pain free. If you see changes or feel he isn't getting what he needs, you call us, and we come right away and help you change the meds and anything else he may need. For now, I'm going to leave you with all the supplies you'll need to care for him and show you a few tricks that will make moving him around for changes and other things much easier on him and on you. I plan to come back at about ten in the morning to tell you how hospice works, what you can expect in the coming days as Rockey moves through this and how we can work together to help him be most comfortable. Does that sound okay to you? Do you have family in the area?"

I answered "Rockey's son Nick lives in Gateway, and his other son is traveling here from Minnesota."

She said, "If they can both be here at 10:00 a.m., that would be best for all of you to hear all the information." I told her I would encourage them to come.

After she left, I thought about her and how she made me feel. She came in with authority, but it didn't feel pushy or aggressive. She was smiley and warm but allowed for some distance. She spoke respectfully to and about Rockey and gave me all the authority for all decisions without saying a word about it. I felt no doubts or hesitations about her medical expertise or the fact that Rockey's case landed in her hands. She moved briskly but not so fast as to be abrupt. It was, I decided, one of the most interesting profiles of the perfect human for this difficult job I could have imagined. She left me feeling confident and calm about my ability to manage the coming storm, and I was beyond grateful that she was on our side.

Delilah hung around until about 8:00 p.m. I told her I would be okay, and she should get home. We had made some food and sort of hung out in the vicinity of Rock's bed, trying not to be so noisy that we disturbed him. He looked to be sleeping, but I thought he was hovering between sleep and wake. Delilah went to his side, laid her hand on his chest and softly said, "Good night, Rock. I'm going home but I'll be back tomorrow. Mag is here and you're in good hands." He reached up slowly and covered her tiny hand with his giant one, never opening his eyes.

He had a fitful night. I was on the couch in another room and every sound he made alerted me. I checked him several times to see if he needed his Depends changed. He did and I was out of my league with the lifting required for the task. It took all my one-armed strength to get the job done and I'm not sure I did an adequate job. If he bumped the bed rail, I jumped up to see if he was trying to rise. He screamed and kicked through some night terrors, and I could only try to comfort him. He was here but not here. I slept not one wink.

The next day started with a flurry of activity. Delilah came and felt like a cool drink on a hot day. She tended to Rock, softly cleaning his face and torso with a wet cloth, speaking in her whispery talk to him. She was able to feed him a bit of yogurt and he greedily drank some water. I was on the phone, still trying to fill out the slim ranks of caregivers. The pandemic had hit that industry hard, and there were very few people available. I knew I wasn't going to be able to keep up my twenty-four-hour watches for long. I had picked up my habit of rubbing my face and pulling on my eyebrow, signs that I was nearly unable to continue. Nick came, bringing his permanently sad brother Rock Jr., and his wife, Angie. Jan came and took us through how Rock would be cared for, what drugs we should give for his pain and to help quiet his broken mind. She was refreshingly honest about dying.

She informed me about the process a body goes through, and I was relieved to have the information and very glad the kids heard the same words. She reminded us that Rockey had almost no control in his life right now, except for what he chose to eat and drink or whether he chose to do so. We were told that everyone on this path eventually stops taking in both food and water as the body begins to shut down. It was our job to offer it to him, and our job to respect his wishes when he refused. I liked the way she presented that. A nurse from hospice would come every other day as would the lovely woman, Janelle, who bathed Rock and gently applied lotion to his skin and dressed him in clean clothes. She offered care tips to make our job easier and more efficient and to make the whole thing less abrupt and invasive for Rockey.

I was continually tested by the chaos that now visited my home. Rockey and I had lived quietly alone for so long, the bodies, the voices, the doors opening, and closing were like screeching to me. I functioned well in our solitude and was quick to understand that even though I needed all this help, the core of me screamed out for silence and less movement. Finally, everyone except Delilah took their leave and I wanted to fall on my knees with gratitude for their absence.

I wasn't eating and had no desire to. An old friend brought us a homemade chicken pot pie and it was good fuel for the helpers. I hadn't grocery shopped for a long while and didn't consider it now. That wonderful tradition of bringing food to people in crisis was something else I was thankful for.

Sometime late in the day, there was a knock at the laundry room door. I opened it to find Rocky Jr and Angie standing there with suitcases. This was Rock's son who hadn't spoken to me in decades and never looked me in the eye. I had about ten seconds to decide whether I would do the right thing for his broken-hearted son and invite the intruders into my home so he could find some peace with his father's dying, or whether I would tell them to leave their bags outside. They had not texted or called to announce their arrival. I hated, really hated, the thought of those two people who never had a kind word for me being in my home around the clock. But I couldn't abide the image I would have of myself for turning them away. I said, "Oh, you're planning to stay?" Jr remained mute, staring at the ground, and Angie said, "We thought we could help." I opened the door and let them in and told them they could have Rockey's bedroom. While they dragged too much luggage through the house, I texted Nick and said, "WTF? Rocky and Angie just showed up with suitcases. I thought they were staying with you."

Nick was aware of my distrust for both of these characters and knew I would not have agreed to them staying here, had I been given a forewarning. He texted back, "Angie can help you. She'll do whatever you ask. Take the help, Mag." I knew he was right, but I still hated it. "They could have fucking called first," I texted back.

Delilah was getting ready to leave and wouldn't be back for a few days. I felt my heart pinch a little as I hugged the only friend I felt I had in this new mess. She was there for Rockey's care, but this tiny woman, barely into her twenties, somehow made me feel protected too.

They hovered around Rockey in a sort of maudlin vigil. I knew if he was conscious, he would hate the hovering. I stayed back in the kitchen to avoid further crowding into Rockey's space. They seemed unaware that, even lying still with his eyes closed, he could comprehend the people and events around him. He was inani mate to them, and it felt undignified to me. I motioned them to the kitchen and told them if they needed to talk about him, do so out of earshot of him. They said, "Well he isn't even awake." I said firmly, "He's in there and he can hear what you're saying. Don't talk about him as if he's not there."

Rockey was getting a small dose of morphine as well as Lorazepam. I resurrected my practice of keeping meticulous records on everything we gave him, including times and amounts dispensed. He wasn't as sedated as I would have expected. Nick's wife, Megan, called and asked if she could bring the kids over. I said, "Absolutely!" They came in and Andi said a timid hello to her rough-looking papa and decided to hang out and play a little distance from Rock. Elliot crawled right up and ran his dump truck up and down Rockey's legs, all the while Rock held his face in an odd, frozen smile. Megan asked if they were being too noisy or too rough for Rock. I said, "Their voices are like music to him, and Elliot is doing nothing but good right now." I left them to themselves and could hear Megan talking softly to Rock. She had great tears in her eyes when she packed the kids up to leave. "I wish I could do more, do something." she said. I told her, "What you just did is the very best thing you could have given him. Time with your kids. Try to come again if you can."

After she left, I found myself in the rare moment where it was just Rockey and me and he was awake. I sat beside him and took his hand. He cried for a little while, saying, "The babies. The babies." Then he said to me, "Overdose?"

I said, "Yes."

He said, "Fucked that up?" Again, I said yes. He lifted his eyebrows as if asking a question and squeezed my hand and said, "Help me?"

I made a sad face and said, "No. I can't help you, Rock. I won't go to jail for you."

He was quiet for a minute, then said, "The ladies."

I asked, "Do you mean the hospice ladies?" He nodded. "They are here to help you. They give you comfort and care. The care is the bathing and taking care of your body for you. The comfort is the drugs. Do you understand?"

He nodded again. He looked me in the eyes and said, "More comfort. Faster please."

I squeezed his hand and said, "Soon enough. It will take however long it takes."

He closed his eyes and whispered, "Faster." Then he was gone again.

That evening, Rockey became restless. He was shuffling his legs and kicking at the covers, grabbing the bed rail, mumbling about having to pee. Angie and Jr were next to him, and Angie was telling him why he couldn't get up and Rock Jr. was reenforcing that he needed to stay in bed. He kicked and fought and bitched and swore and talked nonsense but exhibited surprising strength.

At one point he shouted, "You sonsabitches need to take me home!"

I went over and said, "Rock, you are home." He kicked and shook the rail, and as I sat down beside him on the bed, he swung a fist so fast at my face I felt the wind of it as I pulled my head back. His feet were pulled up, so his knees were in the air, and I backhand slapped his knees lightly and pointed at his face and said, "No hitting, Rock. There will be no hitting." He turned, and amazingly fast, grabbed Rock Jr. by the wrists and just pulled. I could see the pressure on Junior's skin as it blanched white then turned purple around his dad's tight grip. I said, "Rock, what are you doing? That's your son you're hurting now."

Junior said softly, "I'm okay."

They remained there with that horrible hard grip and Big Rock muttering menacingly through his gritted teeth, "Take me home, you fuckers!" He kicked at Angie, and I told her to stay the hell back. I took Big Rock's wrists in my hands and squeezed them, trying to get him to let go of his son, to no avail. Just before this aggressive position, Rockey was whispering intently about it being "Go time. Come on, Jason is waiting." He began reaching and grabbing imaginary things and I asked what he was grabbing, and he said, "The helmets. Get your helmet, now! We're invading their compound." I made the mistake of trying to talk him out of the invasion and that's when he snapped into the aggression towards us.

We stayed in this nasty grip for about a half hour, and I decided a new voice might help. I called his friend Bob and told him we needed help, that Rock was agitated and hurting his kid. Dear Bob walked through the front door within minutes and went to Rockey's bed and sat right down. He said, "Hey pardner, I hear you're having some trouble. What can I do to help you figure this out?" Rock dropped his grip on junior and mumbled something about fire and Bob said, "No, Rock. You know I can see everybody from my house up there and there's no fires tonight. I can promise you that." I couldn't quite hear the next words from Rockey, but it was something about the horse bleeding. Again, Bob said, "Well, I keep a pretty good eye on things around here when you're under the weather. I looked in at the horses when I drove by and they sure are fat and happy, and nobody was bleeding."

Bob didn't look at any of us but kept his focus on his old friend. There was some more talk, and finally Bob stood up and said, "Well, I think we got some things figured out, eh Rock?" Rockey nodded. Bob went on, "Now you have to be a little more agreeable with these kids and Mag; they're just trying to help you get better. And you got to get better because we have stuff to do, Rockey. Okay?" Rock nodded and shook Bob's hand and his eyes teared up. Bob slipped out the front door and was gone. Rockey was quiet the rest of that evening.

After things quieted down and I had a chance to think, I realized this incident was my fault. Rockey had a favorite show about a S.E.A.L. team. He didn't have his eyes open, but I knew he could hear, so I turned on the TV show. In his tossed-salad brain, he moved into the show, became one of the team and acted it out in our living room. A new rule was born from that incident: no TV at all. No electronic sounds were allowed in his area.

I called hospice first thing and told them about his aggression. The nurse had a consult with their on-staff doctor, and they decided that because the pain pump carried morphine, this additional dose was just enough to make Rockey agitated, a common reaction when morphine levels are high. They changed it out for another drug and had it delivered by mid-day. It worked well and his agitation was greatly diminished, but so was his consciousness.

We decided that Angie would take the night shifts, and I would do the day watching. I think Rock Jr. sat with his dad until midnight and then Angie took over. It felt heavenly to go downstairs with my dogs, turn on the television or browse the internet with no yelling or needs or frightening moments. I cracked the window so I could hear the owls and the coyotes calling. The days were finally getting quieter. Rockey stopped eating, and a day or two later, he stopped drinking. We would use a tiny syringe to squirt water into his mouth. His head had fallen to his right side and try as we might we were not able to straighten his neck out as it caused him pain. His right eye, with the old injury on his iris, swelled some and the eye no longer closed. It was freakish looking, and I'm sure made everyone a little uncomfortable. Rock Jr. slept until around 10:00 a.m. Angie was critical about the food philosophy for Big Rock. She thought we should be pleading with him. I explained more than once that it was his choice, and it was a natural progression toward dying. I heard later that she told people I killed him by denying him food. Stupidity is never an excuse for cruelty.

Big Rock's birthday was December 12 and one of the "kids" thought we should have a birthday party for him. I eventually told them that Rock didn't want a birthday party when he was well; he certainly wouldn't want one with people laughing and talking just out of reach of his mind. I offered to give them steaks enough for all, and they should have a party in his honor at Nick's. I think they did because I remember having a little time alone with Rock. During the few times we were left alone, I would sit by his bed and stroke his arm and tell him our stories. I reminded him of our best times or the funniest times or places where our private jokes were born. The time we hiked up Beehive Basin, long before it was a neighborhood, when it was still a lovely forest leading up toward the trail to Spanish Peaks. It was fall, and the golden light shafted through the aspens at a picturesque angle as we hiked steadily higher. I grabbed his hand and pulled him off the trail to a little creek and said, "We should make love right here. Look at it—it's so beautiful!" He looked around and nervously said, "Someone could see us." I pulled him to the ground and said, "We haven't seen another human for hours." As I undid his jeans, I said, "Besides, if I play my cards right, they're only going to see your white ass." When we finished, he stood quickly, pulling up his jeans, and he looked at me and said, "There." I laughed so hard I couldn't even dress. One of us said the same thing at the end of most of our lovemaking for the rest of our days. It still cracked us both up.

I retold the story of Pete the mule running off into the Bob Marshall Wilderness with the other pack mules tied to him when Rockey stepped off to pee. It took us three hours to right that mess. Then there was NM—a naked man who walked through the beach chairs every day when we were learning to scuba dive in the Grand Caymans. The time Pancho got impatient while we unpacked the mules at the high camp in the Porcupine drainage. His good horse untied himself and rolled in the rocks, destroying Rockey's saddle. Rock had spent a lot of words bragging about his good, good horse. I laughed until I cried when he picked up the broken saddle, knowing it would mean he would be walking out leading his good horse. I whispered, "Remember all the sex we had in the model homes? The time you dug up a nest of bees with the bobcat?"

I also told him thank you.

Thank you for those years when you loved me so. I told him I was sorry that he had to live like this. I told him he had been my greatest love.

Delilah came quietly into the room one day when I was telling him stories and later asked, "What is it you're telling him, Mag?" I smiled and said, "I'm trying to fill up his head with goodness. Maybe if I keep layering in the good stories, they will overtake the terrors he sees in his mind. Just trying to help him leave with the memories that were happy." I shrugged, a little embarrassed, as if to say maybe it's dumb, but they are still good stories.

He slipped away from us in these last days. There were no more sounds. No more rustling feet. He couldn't take the few drops of water I offered. They just fell out of his mouth.

I woke up at 5:40 a.m. on Tuesday morning, December 15. I was not startled but was wide awake. I knew he had gone. I made my way upstairs and was glad to be the only one awake. I touched him softly on the face and he was still warm, but he was not here. I wished him fair trails and good travel as I kissed his cheek one last time. I made the phone calls that I needed to make. Hospice would come and make the arrangements for the funeral home and the coroner. I called Nick and woke Angie from her sleep on the couch. I called my sister and asked her to call the others.

Delilah texted and said she was running late. I answered with, "No hurry. Rock is gone." She said, "I'm on my way." She hugged me hard when she came in the door, and I was nearly undone by the comfort of that embrace. The funeral home came quickly, had me fill out some papers, and I specified cremation and they took Rockey away. I did not watch them leave.

Delilah and I walked down the driveway and she asked, "What do you want to do this day, Maggie? I'm staying until you tell me to leave."

I said, "I want to make a fire in the firepit and hang around, drink coffee and tell some Rockey stories. Indians have a great tradition of fire when someone dies and believe that the rising smoke helps them on their journey. I want us to do that."

It was a cold day and, women being so good at taking care of everything, it wasn't long until there was plenty of wood, a couple of chairs around the fire and flames to warm us. I took care of getting strong, hot coffee with plenty of cream. We sat and we stood and stomped our feet to keep warm and told some stories of Rockey. I told some funny stories of our flaming-hot early years and the spontaneous lovemaking here, there and everywhere. While we stood there for a few hours, stoking the fire and talking, Delilah would disappear into the house from time to time, and I never thought much of it. When we agreed we had enough of our very cold feet, Delilah and I went into the house. I found that Delilah's disappearances had been in service to me. She washed all the bedding, all the towels, all his clothes and pushed the hospital bed against a wall, stacking all the leftover supplies and the folded linens neatly on top of it. I was so glad to not have to deal with that mess.

Delilah stayed through the day, her presence like a balm to me. The telephone was mercifully quiet as I took my first steps into life without Rockey.

When the smoke from the western fires no longer chokes us and the temperature dips below unbearably hot, I will saddle up good horse Louie and ride to the place of the high-country camp Rock and I loved for so many summers. I will hope for a breeze to scatter his ashes across the rocks on that ridge where he sat so peacefully and so often. I am old now and that basin is far, but I hope a member from my tiny circle of friends will ride with me and the dogs. What remains of Rockey deserves some peace.

So do I.

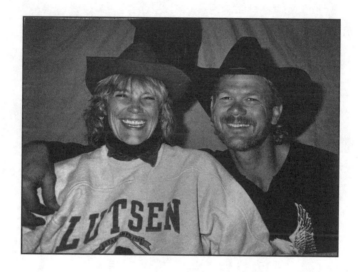

Rock and Maggie, 1994

Acknowledgments

This book was born in my mind the summer of 2014, when everything with Rockey's health went so terribly wrong. After he died in December of 2020, I enrolled in an online writing class that I had previously dropped out of when his needs for care were great. That class and the support and eagle eyes of those students gave me the confidence to dive into this book and see what I could create. Duella Scott- Hull became a true and steadfast friend, encouraging me and routinely calling me to task, through the process of writing. Roz Spafford reminded me often that it was my story too. It was these two who lit the path for me.

Andrea Peacock, Elise Atchison and Maryanne Vollers, who originally motivated me at the first Elk River Writers Workshop, gave me quiet, unwavering support and asked good questions that helped me form a better narrative. Elise's editing skills are among the best in the business. Tracy Pechachek, Kim Chater, Leslie Hayes ... dearest friends to me who carried me through my grief, more often than they will ever know. My deep love and gratitude to my sister Kathy Anderson Olson for everything and for always.

My appreciation is huge for the nurses in all the hospitals who took a moment to touch my shoulder or embrace me, whispering words of strength. Mom, I carried you with me and knew you'd be proud.

Finally, to Daniel Rice, for taking a chance on a rookie author.

Thank you all for believing in my storytelling.

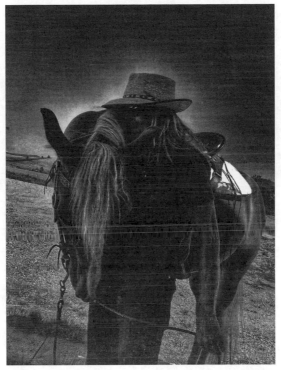
photo by Holly Pippel

Maggie Anderson lives in a beautiful valley in Montana. She continues to hike with her dogs and explore the backcountry with her horse. She is thriving.

Other titles from Riverfeet Press

THIS SIDE OF A WILDERNESS: A Novel —Daniel J. Rice

ECOLOGICAL IDENTITY: Finding Your Place in a Biological World —Timothy Goodwin

ROAD TO PONEMAH: The Teachings of Larry Stillday —Michael Meuers

A FIELD GUIDE TO LOSING YOUR FRIENDS —Tyler Dunning

AWAKE IN THE WORLD, V.1: a collection of stories, poems, and essays about wildlife, adventure, and the environment

ONE-SENTENCE JOURNAL (winner of the 2018 Montana Book Award and the 2019 High Plains Book Award) —Chris La Tray

WILDLAND WILDFIRES: And Where the Wildlife Go —Randie Adams

I SEE MANY THINGS: Ninisidawenemaag, Book I —Erika Bailey-Johnson

AWAKE IN THE WORLD, V.2: a collection of stories, poems, and essays about wildlife, adventure, and the environment

REGARDING WILLINGNESS (2020 Montana Honor Book) —Tom Harpole

BURNT TREE FORK: A Novel —J.C. Bonnell

LIFE LIST: Poems —Marc Beaudin

WITHIN THESE WOODS —Timothy Goodwin

KAYAK CATE —Cate Belleveau

TEACHERS IN THE FOREST —Barry Babcock

THE UNPEOPLED SEASON: Ten Year Anniversary Edition —Daniel J. Rice

WILTED WINGS (2023 Spur Award Finalist) —Mike McTee

BEYOND THE RIO GILA —Scott G. Hibbard

AWAKE IN THE WORLD, V.3: A Riverfeet Press Anthology

www.riverfeetpress.com

PRINTED IN THE USA